CANCER, SICKNESS, AND FAITH:

GOD'S HELP FOR YOU

BY

BOB INGRAM

BLYTHEWOOD, SOUTH CAROLINA

MAY 2023

i

Cover Design by Chippy Miner

ISBN: 979 83 90146743

# TABLE OF CONTENTS

# ACKNOWLEDGMENTS

Nine years ago, when I was faced with cancer, I wasn't afraid, but it got my attention. It made me think about the faith walk that I had heard preached decades before and how it applied to my life. The church I pastored at the time, LifeGate Assembly of God, in Burlington, New Jersey, supported me as I was treated for cancer. They allowed me a three-month Sabbatical as I had a stem-cell transplant and waited on my immune system to recover. For that I am thankful.

LifeGate also listened to my sermons as I preached about many subjects including faith. For seven and a half years they watched me deal with cancer. In September of 2021, I began a new round of treatment with a new drug because my cancer numbers reflected an advancement of the disease. The church still supported me, but shortly after that I resigned, retired, and moved to South Carolina to be with my grandkids. My wife and I love and miss our church family in New Jersey. I will never forget the support they gave me as I pastored them over eleven years.

Since retiring and moving to South Carolina, it has been difficult leaving so many memories we had in Jersey, but having more time has allowed me to continue my quest for understanding living by faith. This book is about my quest. I hope that it helps you.

A special thanks to my editor Cody Smith for helping me write better. He found most of my mistakes, challenged my reasoning, and helped me improve my research.

Thanks to Chippy Miner for the cover design. I have watched her grow from a young child in my kids' choir to an amazing graphic design artist.

Of course, I am so thankful for my wife of 47 years for her support in so many areas throughout our marriage. She is my rock and encourager. She put up with me as I disappeared upstairs to work on writing. She listened to my ideas and offered her comments. Thanks so much for your help.

# CHAPTER 1: INTRODUCTION

In the early 70s, I became acquainted with the faith teaching of people such as Kenneth Copeland, Jerry Seville, Charles Capps, and others. At that time, I had never heard anyone teach about faith and believing in the "Word." I had never read the Bible much and certainly didn't think of the Bible as something that would direct my life. This was the beginning of a new journey for me.

Though I went to church as a kid, I wouldn't consider my home a Christian home. My dad was in the military and an alcoholic. Our home had all the issues that alcoholism brings. When the club closed on the military base, it was not unusual for my dad to bring 20 people home and party at our house until early in the morning. He would wake us up, my mother to play piano and my sister and I to sing, "I have a little candle light." Somehow, my mother kept the family together. She took us to the protestant church services on the military base. I heard about Jesus there, but never understood that a relationship with God was required or desired. Though I learned a few Scriptures, regular Bible reading wasn't encouraged.

In college, I found Jesus, or should I say Jesus found me. I attended a Bible-believing church but didn't regularly read the Bible because no one encouraged me to read it. My senior year in college, I began playing with a gospel group that was based out of a non-denominational church that embraced the "Faith" teaching.[1]    The idea of studying the Bible, carrying it everywhere, and underlining passages was totally new to me.    They memorized Scriptures and even hugged each other at church. I thought they were nuts and they made me uncomfortable. Somehow, I hung around and began reading the Bible. I would memorize whole chapters of the Bible and countless other Scriptures. I was hungry for God.

For the first time, I heard the "Confession is Possession" and "Name it and claim it" doctrine.[2] Though I studied it, I felt that something was missing from the teaching. How could all of someone's problems be attributed to "lack of faith?" Maybe that was true some of the time, but it seemed to me that the "Faith" message didn't include the whole counsel of God's Word. How could God make living by faith so hard that almost no one could live it? It seemed to me that the "Faith" message was shallow and concentrated too much on getting stuff from God and not living obediently for God. To me, it seemed that the success of a believer was measured by the vehicle they drove or where they lived.

Below are a couple of quotes from the website GotQuestions.org. The first one describes their viewpoint. The second quote discusses their view of the prosperity gospel.

---

[1] The "Faith" teaching focused a great deal on the authority a believer has in Christ and the blessing that God wants to give you. It also emphasized the importance of a person's verbal confession to bringing change in one's life.

[2] Kenneth Hagin along with others started the "Faith" teaching which included the idea that what you say matters and can change things.

*GotQuestions.org is a ministry of dedicated and trained servants who have a desire to assist others in their understanding of God, Scripture, salvation, and other spiritual topics. We are Christian, Protestant, evangelical, theologically conservative, and non-denominational. We view ourselves as a para-church ministry, coming alongside the church to help people find answers to their spiritually related questions.*

*We will do our best to prayerfully and thoroughly research your question and answer it in a biblically based manner. It is not our purpose to make you agree with us, but rather to point you to what the Bible says concerning your question. You can be assured that your question will be answered by a trained and dedicated Christian who loves the Lord and desires to assist you in your walk with Him. Our writing staff includes pastors, youth pastors, missionaries, biblical counselors, Bible/Christian college students, seminary students, and lay students of God's Word.[3]*

Here is the second quote describing *Gotquestions.org* definition of the Word of Faith Movement.

*In the prosperity gospel, also known as the "Word of faith movement" the believer is told to use God, whereas the truth of biblical Christianity is just the opposite—God uses the believer. Prosperity theology sees the Holy Spirit as a power to be put to use for whatever the believer wills. The Bible teaches that the Holy Spirit is a Person who enables the believer to do God's will. The prosperity gospel movement closely resembles some of the destructive greed*

---

[3] "About Got Questions.Org", Got Questions.org, accessed Oct. 14, 2022, https://www.gotquestions.org/about.html.

*sects that infiltrated the early church. Paul and the other apostles were not accommodating to or conciliatory with the false teachers who propagated such heresy. They identified them as dangerous false teachers and urged Christians to avoid them.[4]*

Gotquestions.org is led by S. Michael Houdmann who has a conservative Baptist background and therefore not inherently positive towards a Pentecostal perspective, of which the Faith Movement is a part.[5]

However, I believe he is correct in pointing out that the Prosperity Gospel focuses on what God can do for you or what you can do for yourself through your faith rather than a life lived in obedience to God's will. In fact, the Prosperity Gospel would say that it is God's will for you to live in victory in all areas of your life including financially and health wise.

Unfortunately, many American Christians have fallen into the trap of seeing possessions as an indication of God's favor. This has led some to buy things and overextend themselves on credit. The thinking is "I am a child of the King and I deserve the best." The Prosperity Gospel doesn't work as well in developing nations, though often the leadership prospers from it greatly in America and other nations. Truly living by faith involves more than "stuff" or money. It requires obedience and willingness to be

---

[4] "What does the Bible say about the prosperity gospel?", Got Questions.org, accessed Oct. 14, 2022, https://www.gotquestions.org/prosperity-gospel.html.

[5] Baptist theology typically believes in dispensationalism that places modern society in an era that doesn't require the gifts of the Spirit and the Baptism in the Spirit. They base that in part on the Scripture found in 1 Cor. 13 stating, "But when that which is perfect is come, then that which is in part shall be done away" (1 Cor. 13:10 KJV).

used, in addition to willingness to take a "step of faith". More about a step of faith later.

A car wreck took me out of the gospel group and away from that church.[6] God led me to another ministry, where I would eventually meet my future wife. Understanding the "Faith" message was put on the back burner. I continued living for God and studying the Word of God in seminary, but I didn't focus on the "Faith" message. Seminary brought a whole host of new challenges as I learned about the process that brought us our modern-day translations. The more I learned, it seemed the less I knew. There was so much to learn about correctly understanding the Bible and interpreting it correctly, such as studying the original languages of Greek and Hebrew, textual criticism, hermeneutics, cultural and geographic issues, systematic theology, etc.

Surprisingly, prior to attending seminary, in 1978, God lead me into aviation. I had no idea where God was taking me, but I started the process of learning to fly and getting all my ratings. I began my 31-year flying career while in seminary.[7] In 2008, the Lord directed me to renew my ministerial credentials and begin applying for jobs as a lead pastor. I began pastoring LifeGate Assembly of God in 2010 while still flying for the airlines.[8] In 2012, I retired from the airlines and began pastoring fulltime. A year and a

---

[6] Go to Appendix A to read Pastor Bob's testimony.
[7] Go to Appendix B to read about Pastor Bob's adventure into aviation.
[8] Full Gospel Fellowship church was changed to LifeGate Assembly of God in 2016.

half after that, I was diagnosed with multiple myeloma cancer for which there is no cure outside of God.[9]

As I said before, hearing the diagnosis of cancer, didn't strike fear in my life, but it was a wakeup call to my faith and understanding what I really believe. This book is about my adventure of learning to walk by faith. I wrote it to help me in my walk with Jesus. It is my prayer that it will encourage you to seek God with your whole heart and allow the King of Kings and Lord of Lords to empower you to go beyond yourself and live by faith. I will not answer all your questions and may bring up many more questions about your faith that will require you to dig into the Word of God for answers.

I have broken the book down into four sections. Section One looks at Hebrews 11:6 for a definition of faith. Section Two looks at the life of Abraham, the Father of faith. Section Three looks at Mark 11: 22-26, a foundational Scripture for the Prosperity Gospel. Section Four looks at Matthew chapters 8 and 9 to see what Jesus says and does about healing. Don't be afraid to make notes in your Bible. It is your textbook. Join me in this adventure and let's get started.

---

[9] June 18, 2021, I was hit from behind on my motorcycle. I am currently recovering from the accident. The bike was totaled and though no bones were broken; I am dealing with a number of physical issues. Additionally, the myeloma cancer advanced and I begin a new round of chemo in September 2021. This is part of my ongoing faith story. Also because of the combination of cancer treatment and the motorcycle accident, I retired from pastoring in November 2021 at age 70.

# SECTION ONE: DEVELOPING FAITH

## CHAPTER 2: UNDERSTANDING FAITH

Over 45 years ago when I began listening to the "Faith" message, it inspired me, confused me, and disturbed me all at once. It inspired me to read my Bible. For the first time, I was around people that studied the Bible and believed that somehow the promises found in the Word of God worked for them. They talked about healing and living by faith. Wow, I wondered, was it possible?

It confused me because I saw many sick people that didn't get healed, so-called Christians that lived with sickness just like the world. Why did some get healed, and others didn't? Was the person doing something wrong? Was there sin in his or her life that hindered the person's prayers? Was it lack of faith? Were there hindrances outside of them of which they were totally unaware? Was it spiritual warfare? These were some of the questions I had, and I am still learning the answers.

It disturbed me because it seemed that few could live up to that standard that the "Faith Message" preached. I saw some completely lose their faith and walk away when things didn't work as they thought they should. It also disturbed me that often a blessing was based on giving to a certain ministry. As a new Christian, I learned quickly to compare what was preached against what happened in the New Testament church, as recorded in the Book of Acts. I saw nothing in Scripture that indicates you should give to a particular ministry in order to receive the blessings of God.

Also, does what is being preached work in developing nations or is it an American gospel? How do you explain mature Christians having bad things happen to them? Is it lack of faith, or is the "Faith" gospel missing something. These are tough questions, but there are answers.

Jesus' actions also give us direction in our understanding of living by faith. There are countless passages about healings, but everyone doesn't get healed during Jesus' time. The Bible does say that everyone Jesus prayed for was healed, but Jesus didn't pray for everyone. Faith affected Jesus' ability to pray. In the gospel of Matthew, Jesus returns home to people that have a hard time believing He was anything special. Matthew writes,

*[57] And they took offense at him.*

*But Jesus said to them, "A prophet is not without honor except in his own town and in his own home."*
*[58] And he did not do many miracles there because of their lack of faith* (Matt. 13:57-58).[10]

Jesus, the creator of the universe, was limited by people's lack of faith. Whether we want to admit it or not, whether we like it or not, faith or lack of faith affects the outcome of prayer and healing. Jesus confirms this in numerous other Scriptures, including Matthew 8 &9, where He deals with

---

[10] All Scriptures references are NIV unless otherwise noted.

so many questions about healing. We will look more at this in Chapter 12, but first, let's define faith.

## Defining Faith

### Believe God exists

The author of Hebrews writes, "And without faith it is impossible to please God, because anyone who comes to him must believe that he exists and that he rewards those who earnestly seek him" (Heb. 11:6). Notice that faith is required to please God. The author continues defining faith as believing in the existence of God. This may seem like an easy thing to do, but we live in a society that is anti-God and attempts to legislate Him out of existence. Recent statistics show the number of people that believe in God, any god, is decreasing.

> *The vast majority of U.S. adults believe in God, but the 81% who do so is down six percentage points from 2017 and is the lowest in Gallup's trend. Between 1944 and 2011, more than 90% of Americans believed in God. Gallup's May 2-22 Values and Beliefs poll finds 17% of Americans saying they do not believe in God.*[11]

Still, the first step to faith is to believe that God exists. How do we do that? The Apostle Paul tells us that creation tells us about God. "For since

---

[11] Jeffery M. Jones, "Belief in God in U.S. Dips to 81%, a New Low," Gallup.com, June 17, 2022, https://news.gallup.com/poll/393737/belief-god-dips-new-low.aspx.

the creation of the world God's invisible qualities—his eternal power and divine nature—have been clearly seen, being understood from what has been made, so that people are without excuse" (Rom. 1:20).

The writer of Hebrews describes the role of creation. "By faith we understand that the universe was formed at God's command, so that what is seen was not made out of what was visible" (Heb. 11:3). What we believe about creation is foundational to our faith in God. We look at everything differently when we recognize that in the beginning, God created the heavens and the earth like it tells us in Genesis 1. God gives us purpose and reason for living when He put His image inside of us. But since we weren't there, we must take it by faith.

We can't see God, but that doesn't mean that we can't see His handwork. Just look around at God's creation. God's creation is too complex, too big, too small, too beautiful, and too varied to just have happened. Evolution wants us to believe that things just evolved over millions and millions of years, but creation shouts against that idea.

Think about the incredible ability of the human eye. It can see in such a wide range of light and can focus up close and far away. The eye's ability to see so many colors is remarkable. There have been huge advances in TV, film production, computers, cameras, and smart phones attempting to see as well as the human eye does. Humanity wants to give credit to men and women for the engineering and computer science accomplishments but somehow it is accepted that something far more complex than anything that humanity has designed, the human body for example, just happened. It

17

evolved. That is nonsense. Creation screams at us there is a loving, powerful, creative God that wants us to know Him.

There are so many other things in the human body that tells us God designed it. Think about the human cell, for example, which has a nucleus in the middle of it. The nucleus is like the office of the cell. It contains the DNA which is the blueprint for the cell. If a copy is needed of the DNA, the cell makes a copy, the RNA molecule, that is sent out of the nucleus.[12] The whole process of the reproduction of the human cells is too complex to have evolved.

For over 60 years scientists have studied DNA and have made phenomenal progress in unlocking the secrets of it, but DNA is just a small part of the human cell. For example, proteins play an important role in the operation of the cell. One function is to act like custom agents controlling the entrance and exit of molecules into the country (cell).[13] The complexity and design of the human cell make it beyond the realm of chance to have simply happened. It shows the hand of God in creation.

The human blood gives us huge amounts of data about how our bodies are doing. Each time I get my blood checked for cancer treatment, there are over 50 parameters that are looked at. One time, I was visiting a congregant at the University of Penn neurology ward and noticed on the wall a diagram showing parts of the human brain. I tried to memorize the

---

[12] Rene Fester Kratz, *Molecular and Cell Biology for Dummies* (Hoboken, NJ: Wiley Publishing, Inc., 2009), 22.
[13] Kratz, 17.

18

names while I waited. I couldn't. It was too complex. Evolution wants to say it just happened. Not possible.

There is plenty of evidence to prove that God exists. Our world, including outer space, tells us that there is a God. Humanity chooses to ignore it because knowing there is a God means that there is accountability. It also means that God could have an opinion about how we live our lives. Most people don't want to obey God so denying God's existence for a time seems to resolve the internal conflict.

That brings us to the second part of Hebrews 11:6. "And without faith it is impossible to please God, because anyone who comes to him must believe that he exists and that he rewards those who earnestly seek him". There are a couple of key points to consider here. First, God rewards. Second, He rewards those that earnestly seek Him, which we will talk about later in the section "Earnestly Seeks." God blesses those that seek Him. God intervenes in their lives. Does that mean He will make you a millionaire? No. Remember, the gospel is not just an American gospel. The gospel is the good news for Cambodia, or Kenya, or Ethiopia, or El Salvador or Iran or Ukraine.

The good news or being blessed by God is more than money. God rewards in eternity for sure, but He does reward here as well. It can be healing, help with our family, a job, protection, or so many other things that we take for granted. We can't equate only money with God's blessings. God does reward in tangible ways. God can reward monetarily in this lifetime, but the key is to recognize God as the source of all blessings.

But sometimes the end result is not during our lifetime. Hebrews 11 says that Noah built the ark because God told him to build it. "By faith Noah, when warned about things not yet seen, in holy fear built an ark to save his family. By his faith he condemned the world and became heir of the righteousness that is in keeping with faith" (Heb. 11:7). But in Abraham's situation, God told him his descendants would receive the Promised Land. He didn't get to see it. The author of Hebrews talks about an attitude of faith that is not wrapped up in this life.

> [13] *All these people were still living by faith when they died. They did not receive the things promised; they only saw them and welcomed them from a distance, admitting that they were foreigners and strangers on earth.* [14] *People who say such things show that they are looking for a country of their own.* [15] *If they had been thinking of the country they had left, they would have had opportunity to return.* [16] *Instead, they were longing for a better country—a heavenly one. Therefore God is not ashamed to be called their God, for he has prepared a city for them* (Heb. 11:13-16).

When you hear a gospel preached that is only about this life and the rewards of this life, run. It is not the full gospel of God. This life is so short. It doesn't even represent a small percent of our life when compared with eternity.

The author of Hebrews lists people that saw the results of their faith and many that didn't.

> *There were others who were tortured, refusing to be released so that they might gain an even better*

*resurrection. [36] Some faced jeers and flogging, and even chains and imprisonment. [37] They were put to death by stoning; they were sawed in two; they were killed by the sword. They went about in sheepskins and goatskins, destitute, persecuted and mistreated—[38] the world was not worthy of them. They wandered in deserts and mountains, living in caves and in holes in the ground.*

*[39] These were all commended for their faith, yet none of them received what had been promised, [40] since God had planned something better for us so that only together with us would they be made perfect* (Heb. 11:35b-40).

As you can see from the last part of this chapter, things didn't go so well, from an earthly standpoint, because some didn't receive their reward in this lifetime. When things don't go the way we hoped, we need to have faith in God that He has everything under control. Faith and hope are not only about this life. We must get an eternal perspective. If you live to be 100 years old, that is nothing compared to the time we will have in eternity. Our faith and hope should be geared towards eternity, not simply having things happen during this lifetime. We often do not see God's eternal perspective.

We live in a world system that stands in opposition to God's Word, challenging us to doubt it with contradictory thoughts. We need to renew our minds through God's Word to grasp how we should live in this world.

A couple more things about the Romans passage that was mentioned earlier. The Apostle Paul writes,

*18 The wrath of God is being revealed from heaven*
*against all the godlessness and wickedness of people, who*
*suppress the truth by their wickedness, 19 since what may be*
*known about God is plain to them, because God has made it*
*plain to them. 20 For since the creation of the world God's*
*invisible qualities—his eternal power and divine nature—have*
*been clearly seen, being understood from what has been made,*
*so that people are without excuse*
(Rom. 1:18-20).

I have underlined a couple of things critical to our understanding of how God works and how He relates to humanity. We <u>can know</u> God is real. That is what God's Word says. God has made it plain to us through "What has been made" or His creation. We can know about God's invisible qualities through creation. The problem is not our ability to know God, but our lack of desire to know God.

What happens when we reject knowing God? It causes the progression of sin to continue. We see that as continue reading Romans 1. Scripture tells us that although they knew God was real, they refused to recognize Him. Because of this, it says that "God gave them over" in verse 24, 26, and 28. In another words, God said, "You want it, you got it." Their minds became depraved.

Each step farther away from God causes more problems. Many of these problems are related to sexual impurity. We see that in our society today. The aggressive gay agenda is a direct result of sin. The norm of living together without getting married is another example. Also, the last statement I highlighted was about them approving of others participating in their sin.

Our society has gotten more promiscuous, and actions once considered private are boldly displayed in public. Our society encourages and often endorses sinful behavior.

To please God, we must join the group that believes God exists and wants to know Him. Also, according to the passage in Hebrews 11, we must believe that God rewards those that earnestly seek Him. So, the beginning of the faith walk involves believing that God exists and choosing to earnestly seek Him.

It is important to know that if living for God is new for you, God takes you where you are at today. He doesn't condemn you for your past sins but begins a work in you from where you are today. Put aside anything that is keeping you from living for God and give Him your life. That means accepting Jesus as Lord and Savior of your life. There is more about salvation on page 32.

The Word of God

Let me insert here a key point about our adventure into understanding faith in God. Certainly, our own experiences influence our relationship with God. However, we should not let our experiences define or limit what God can do. If we need to look beyond our experiences to find and grow in our relationship, then what do we use to guide us? The short answer is the Word of God or the Bible. If you don't believe that the Bible is the Word of God, then it will be difficult for you to have a structure and basis for your faith. Let's look at a couple of key Scriptures that define how we should view Scripture.

The Apostle Paul writes, "[16] All Scripture is God-breathed and is useful for teaching, rebuking, correcting and training in righteousness, [17] so that the servant of God may be thoroughly equipped for every good work" (2 Tim. 3:16-17). When we view God's Word, the Bible, with the proper attitude, it helps us change. We compare our lives with what the Word of God says about us.

Many misunderstand the process that God used to bring about the Bible. Often people will say, "I don't believe the Bible is the Word of God because it is written by man." It is absolutely true that the Bible was written by man, but that makes the process more powerful. To understand what I mean, let me add some thoughts about what it means to be "inspired" or "God-breathed."

When an Old Testament prophet, such as Isaiah, wrote something down, he was inspired by God. God didn't dictate to the prophet the words to say, but "breathed" into him His message. The prophet wrote God's message down using his own vocabulary, language, and style of writing. In this case, when Isaiah was done, the Scripture said exactly what God wanted it to say. However, often the prophet did not know about what he was writing.

For example, when Isaiah was writing about the crucifixion of Jesus in Isaiah 53, crucifixion hadn't been invented yet. He might have understood certain aspects of the passage, but God had inspired him to write

24

for future generations, even though Isaiah didn't understand everything about which he was writing.

Once the Scriptures were written, the Hebrew scribes went through a laborious procedure to make additional copies. Samuel J. Schultz, when he wrote *The Old Testament Speaks*, was a professor of Old Testament at Tampa Bay Theological Seminary and professor emeritus of Bible and Theology at Wheaton College. He writes, "The scholars peculiarly devoted to this task in subsequent centuries were known as Masoretes. They copied the text with great care and in time even numbered the verses, words, and letters of each book."[14]

The accuracies of manuscripts were confirmed with the discovery of the Dead Sea Scrolls in 1947. The classic Bible College Text Book, *Exploring the Old Testament* says, "Careful examination by archaeologists and datings made by the Carbon 14 method have led to the conclusion that these writings come from the first or more probably the second century before Christ."[15] Prior to their discovery of the Dead Sea Scrolls, the oldest surviving Scriptures from the Old Testament dated to around AD 900. The Dead Sea Scrolls are dated at approximately 100 BC and proved the accuracy of the transmission of the Old Testament Scriptures.[16]

---

[14] Samuel J. Schultz, *The Old Testament Speaks: A Complete Survey of Old Testament History and Literature*, 4th ed. (San Francisco: Harper and Row,1990), 2-3.
[15] W.T. Purkiser, ed. and C.E. Damaray, Donald S. Metz, and Maude A. Stuneck, *Exploring the Old Testament* (Kansas City, MO: Beacon Hill Press, 1955), 63.
[16] Ibid.

The New Testament process is far more complicated. Imagine what it much have been like to receive a letter from the Apostle Paul. When it was received, everyone read it and then copies were made. As the copies were made, the lack of procedures and disciplines like the Jewish Masoretes used allowed for there to be many variant readings. The field of textual criticism examines the manuscripts to find the most accurate one. There are over 5300 manuscripts made from at least 3 materials.

Everett F. Harrison, a missionary and Bible professor, in his *Introduction to the New Testament*, gives us more information about the process. He tells us around 100 A.D. the codex or book form began to be used.[17] That brought up the issue of what was considered Scripture because there were many more writings than what is in today's Bible. Also, decisions had to be made about the order of the books. Marcion, considered a heretic by the early church, came up with his own list and order of canonical books. Think of a canon as a measuring stick. It is a way to determine if a book measures up to what one considers to be Scripture. Marcion had a canon that included only Luke of the gospels and ten Epistles of Paul. Church leadership did not like that, so they solidified their own list of canonical books.[18]

Harrison writes, "It is reasonably certain that the list of New Testament books contained herein was drawn up in conscious opposition to

---

[17] Everett F. Harrison, *Introduction to the New Testament* (Grand Rapids, MI: WM. B. Eerdmans, 1982), 64-65.
[18] Ibid., 103-104.

the canon of the heretic Marcion, whose theological views were unacceptable to the church at Rome."[19] Harrison comments about the influence of later church councils on recognition of Scripture. He continues,

> *It has sometimes been asserted that the canon derives both its form and authority from church councils, as through the church had no recognized Scripture prior to their action. Such is not the case. What the councils did was to certify the canon that was already widely acknowledged in the church.*[20]

Much more could be said about the field of textual criticism but let me sum it up this way. Scholars have devoted their lives over hundreds of years to give us accurate translations in many languages. We can trust the translations. The biggest challenge for us is making sure that we study God's Word and take the time to learn what it says.

The Apostle Paul writes, [15] "Do your best to present yourself to God as one approved, a worker who does not need to be ashamed and who correctly handles the word of truth" (2 Tim. 2:15). Paul emphasized two things that need to be considered. First, we need to present ourselves to God as workers. It takes effort to live for God and it takes effort to study the Word of God.

Second, Paul mentions correctly handling the Word of God. The church is full of false and pet doctrines that people use to tickle their ears, rather than digging in to correctly determine what the Word says. The Word

---

[19] Ibid., 103.
[20] Ibid., 109.

needs to be studied in context of a whole book such as the Book of Ephesians, for example, and then in light of the rest of the writings of that individual author, the Apostle Paul, in this case. Then the whole counsel of the Bible needs to be considered, including the Old Testament. It takes time and effort to learn what the Word of God says. Reading just one passage out of context can glean bad theology.

One more Scripture spreads some light on our journey. "[12] For the word of God is alive and active. Sharper than any double-edged sword, it penetrates even to dividing soul and spirit, joints and marrow; it judges the thoughts and attitudes of the heart" (Heb. 4:12). The Word of God speaks to us and guides us if we let it, but it takes time, effort, and an open heart to receive what God wants to do with our lives.

Earnestly Seek

Back to our second point from Hebrews 11:6, we understand that God rewards those that earnestly seek Him. What does "earnestly seek" mean? Ultimately God decides, but I think that diligently seeking Him is more than attending church every now and then and saying a daily prayer. In my opinion, diligently seeking God should include daily Bible reading and study, plus taking time to meditate on Scriptures and allowing the Holy Spirit the opportunity to speak to us and help us apply the Scriptures to our lives. Also, it includes praying for others and believing that God hears our prayers. It helps to have a system of studying Scriptures so that one does not leave out areas of the Bible that can help us grow.

Unfortunately, many Christians don't read and study the Word of God. Jeremy Weber of Christianity Today writes,

> *One in five of all American adults have read the Bible from start to finish. While it might not be shocking to discover well over half (61%) of evangelical Christians have read the Bible from start to finish, it may be surprising that nearly one in six (18%) of people with a faith other than Christianity and about one in eleven (9%) people with no faith claimed to have done the same. Approximately one-third of politically conservative adults say they have read the Bible, compared with one-tenth of political liberals. Nearly one-third (29%) of black adults say they've read the Bible from start to finish, more than Hispanic adults (22%) and white adults (19%).[21]*

It is not surprising that many Christians don't understand the Word of God because so few have read it, let alone studied it. Jesus understood the difficulties that life brings and the constant stress on one's time. Despite that, He challenges us to keep God first when He says, "But seek first his kingdom and his righteousness, and all these things will be given to you as well" (Matt. 6:33). All the stuff that we worry about will be taken care of if we put God first and diligently seek Him.

Let me add a practical lesson about how God works in our daily lives when we seek Him first. At this moment, I am sitting in a car dealership waiting on an oil change. This is the first since my wife and I bought a used

---

[21] Jeremy Weber, "Surprising Starts on Who Reads the Bible from Start to Finish," Christianity Today, June 4, 2013, https://www.christianitytoday.com/news/2013/june/surprising-stats-on-who-reads-bible-from-start-to-finish.html.

4-year-old car, which was certified, whatever that means. When I showed up, the agent informed me that an oil change wasn't needed for another 5000 miles, and I would have to pay for it if I wanted it. Then he gave me a list of services, totaling about $800 that I thought should be covered by the service agreement I bought when I purchased the car.

Instead of getting upset, I looked to the Lord to help me. Normal daily life is exactly where Jesus helps us. He gets down where we live, whatever we are dealing with, and helps us, whether it is the perceived dishonesty of the dealer, the problems of your boss, or the stock market crash that has happened the last few days, God is still on the throne. He is doing more than answering prayer. If we listen, His Spirit is giving us wisdom to live life. That doesn't mean there will not be challenges. In my case, as the oil change scenario played out, I talked to the general manager and voiced my complaint. It turns out that the dealer is owned by Christians and the GM is a Christian. We were able to discuss the situation and resolve it. Praise God.

Talking about an oil change may seem insignificant and petty in light of the terrible things that are happening today in Ukraine. People there are losing everything they own, their homes, their jobs, their cities, and their families, and they don't know where they are going to live, where their next meal is coming from, or where family members are. War is terrible and I should have nothing to complain about. We are encouraged to pray for situations around the world. Regardless of what is going on in other people's lives and situations around the world, we need to know that God is big enough to handle them and help us with our problems, no matter how small.

Remember the Scripture says we can't please God without faith which requires us to believe He exists and rewards. Does He only reward if your situation is bad enough? No. God is unlimited and is able to help us wherever we live.

The author of Hebrews says that God will reward those that diligently seek Him. The word for rewards, *misthapodotes,* is only used twice in the NT, both in Heb. 10 and 11. Does it mean rewarded in this life? Remember Jesus told us to put God first and not worry about the things of this life and the other stuff will be taken care of. It has to do with priorities, motives, and faith in God. Putting God first in our lives allows Him to work in our lives better than someone that doesn't give God priority. In another words, God will reward you in this life.

*Salvation Explained*

Let me pause here to explain salvation a little bit. We don't get to heaven because we are good enough. In fact, the Bible tells us that none of us are good enough to get to heaven. The Apostle Paul writes, "[23] For all have sinned and fall short of the glory of God, [24] and all are justified freely by his grace through the redemption that came by Christ Jesus" (Rom. 3:23-24). We have all sinned or not measured up to God's standard. That causes a problem between us and God. Since God is perfect, then He has to deal with law-breakers, which is what we are. We have broken His laws and

31

must pay the penalty. Paul writes, "²³ For the wages of sin is death, but the gift of God is eternal life in Christ Jesus our Lord" (Rom. 6:23).

The first passage says that we are "justified freely by his grace through the redemption that came by Christ Jesus." The second passage says, "The gift of God is eternal life." Simply said, Jesus paid our debt, not just for you and me, but for the entire world. There's a catch, however. Paul explains,

> *⁹ If you declare with your mouth, "Jesus is Lord," and believe in your heart that God raised him from the dead, you will be saved. ¹⁰ For it is with your heart that you believe and are justified, and it is with your mouth that you profess your faith and are saved"* (Rom. 10:9-10).

Even though salvation is a gift from God, there is something we have to do. Paul breaks it down into two parts: believing and confessing. What do you believe? That Jesus is the Christ, the Son of the Living God and He arose from the dead. It wouldn't do any good to believe in a dead god. Jesus is alive and sitting at the right hand of the Father and serves there as our high priest interceding on our behalf.

So, to be saved, you have to believe that He is alive. Believing He is the Son of God is not enough, however. James, the brother of Jesus writes, "You believe that there is one God. Good! Even the demons believe that— and shudder" (James 2:19). Believing is more that acknowledging the existence of Jesus as the Son of God, but accepting Him as Lord of your life. The boss of your life. You can read about my salvation experience in Appendix A.

Believing in your heart is not the end of the story. We have to profess or confess that Jesus is Lord. There are no secret disciples. Jesus wants us to tell others about Him. So, the question is where are you today? Is Jesus Lord and Savior of your life? I made that decision over 50 years ago and have never been sorry. In my adventure through cancer, God has greatly helped me. I hope that you will allow Him to be Lord and Savior of your life and help you through your troubles.

To continue our adventure, let's look at the life of the Father of Faith, Abraham, to see what we can learn from him. We will see that in the midst of challenges, he did not always believe that God could work on his behalf.

# SECTION TWO: THE LIFE OF ABRAHAM

## CHAPTER 3: ABRAHAM PART ONE

Abraham is important for us to study, because he is considered the "Father of Faith." As we study his life, we will find principles that apply to ordinary living as well as challenges such as cancer.

God told Abraham to go. "The LORD had said to Abram[22], 'Go from your country, your people and your father's household to the land I will show you'" (Gen. 12:1). God didn't even tell Abraham where he was going, just to go. This brings up a foundational quality of the faith-life: obedience. It isn't about what I want, but what God wants. Many people want the power of faith without the commitment and obedience, but they go hand in hand.

Next God would make promises to Abraham.

> *"I will make you into a great nation, and I will bless you;*
> *I will make your name great, and you will be a blessing.*
> *I will bless those who bless you, and whoever curses you I*
> *will curse;*
> *and all peoples on earth will be blessed through you"*

---

[22] God would later change Abram's name to Abraham (Gen. 17:5). I will refer to Abram as Abraham.

(Gen. 12:2-3).

Abraham would have the ultimate legacy: enough descendants to form a nation and a great name. God promised blessings in five ways:

- God will bless Abraham.
- Abraham will bless others.
- God will bless those that bless Abraham.
- All the people of the earth will be blessed through Abraham.
- God will curse anyone that curses him.

If you look around the world, God's prediction has come true. The Jewish people have a strong presence in the banking industry, the medical field, the movie industry, and the jewelry business, to name a few. Shani Ferguson, a writer for Kehila News, highlights seven ways that Israel and the Jewish people have influenced the world; Medical, humanitarian, social, arts, high tech, security, and spiritual.[23] She writes

*Life-saving products such as WoundClot bandages help compress and clot large wounds, allowing more time to get the patient to a hospital. And with the recent accolades Hadassah Hospital in Jerusalem has received for its da Vinci Robot—which is so precise it can perform brain and spinal surgery with minimally invasive procedures—it is evident that science fiction is just where our scientists go to get ideas for their next invention.[24]*

[23] Shani Ferguson, "Seven ways Israel has impacted your world," Kehila News, July 12, 2018, https://news.kehila.org/seven-ways-israel-has-impacted-your-world/.
[24]Ibid.

Ferguson's article gives many more examples of the vast influence of the Jewish people. The fulfillment of "All the people of the earth will be blessed through Abraham" was Jesus' crucifixion and resurrection.

The following graph is from Pew Research Center. It shows that about one-third of the world population is considered Christian. Notice that the smallest group listed is Jewish.[25] Though tiny in number, the Jewish population has remained front and center in world affairs.

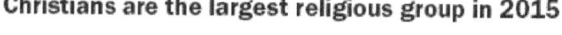

**Christians are the largest religious group in 2015**

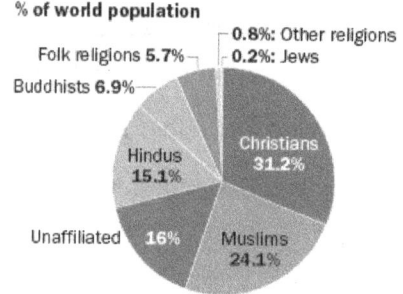
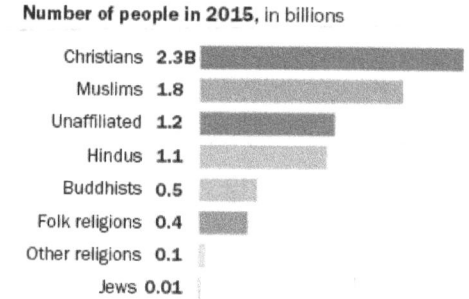

Source: Pew Research Center demographic projections. See Methodology for details. "The Changing Global Religious Landscape"

PEW RESEARCH CENTER

The faith walk that Abraham began when he headed for the Land of Canaan was filled with challenges. The Apostle Paul reminds us that Abraham believed God and it was credited to him as righteousness (Rom.4:3). The Bible shows us the problems that Abraham had walking the

---

[25] Conrad Hackett and David McClendon, "Christians remain world's largest religious group, but they are declining in Europe," Pew Research Center, Washington, D.C. April 5,2017, https://www.pewresearch.org/fact-tank/2017/04/05/christians-remain-worlds-largest-religious-group-but-they-are-declining-in-europe/.

faith walk. This should encourage us because Abraham wasn't a superhuman guy that none of us can hope to emulate. Look at a few points about his life:

| Scripture | Event | Result |
|---|---|---|
| Gen. 12:1-4 | God sends to Abraham to the Land of Canaan. | Abraham was obedient. |
| Gen. 12: 10-20 | Famine in land. | Abraham leaves Canaan and goes to Egypt. Lies about his wife. (See Section: Famine in the Land) |
| Gen. 14 | Abraham demonstrates great courage and rescues his nephew Lot. | He didn't accept payment for rescuing the people. |
| Gen. 15 | God confirms His covenant. | Abraham believes Him. |
| Gen. 16 | Sarah offers Hagar, her slave, to have a child with Abraham. | Abraham has a son, Ishmael, through Hagar. (See Section: Ishmael) |

### Famine in the land

One of the challenges that all of us face is believing that God can work on our behalf in our daily lives, especially when things go wrong, like being diagnosed with cancer. Even though Abraham had dreams and visions from God and maybe even heard His voice, there is no indication that God communicated with him daily any different than you or me. Scripture indicates that Abraham went for years without a message from God. Not hearing from God required Abraham to make decisions on his own. Remember, he had no Bible or church to encourage him.

Let's review what God told Abraham. God told him to "Go" without telling him "Where" to go. When he arrived in the Land of Canaan, God told him to stay. God promised to give the land to his offspring (Gen. 12: 7) which would imply that God would give him offspring and provide for and protect them.

Abraham makes his first mistake when there was a famine, and he left the Promised Land (Gen. 12:10). God didn't tell him to leave. I believe he was supposed to stay in the Promised Land. It takes faith to stay put during a trial. Abraham was showing that he didn't believe that God could provide for him during a famine. It is a challenge for all of us to believe that God can meet our needs when all the evidence is to the contrary. Let me share my own personal experiences with leaving the Promised Land.

Bob leaves the Promised Land the first time

In 1975, I started working for a Christian drug rehabilitation program called Teen Challenge. God called me into this ministry, even though I had never been drunk or used drugs. My dad was an alcoholic. I saw plenty of drunks around the house and didn't want anything to do with drinking or drugs. But God called me to this ministry with people that had problems with alcohol and drugs.

After being at Teen Challenge for about 8 months, I took a trip to Hot Springs, Arkansas to visit some old friends at my former church. This was the church I spoke about earlier that had the gospel group for which I played. I took a bus from Little Rock to Hot Springs because I didn't have a car since I had totaled it. A friend picked me up at the bus station and on the way to a Bible study, stopped at a drug rehab program that the church supported. I watched my friend nail up the front door. The director of the program had backslid and returned to heroin, and they had to shut the program down.

At the Bible study that night, I prayed about that program. I asked the Lord if He wanted me to quit Teen Challenge and run that program. In the spirit, I heard the answer, "Move the Men's home to Hot Springs." Because of the way my mind works, I could see the issues involved with moving the home to Hot Springs, such as funding, leadership and staffing, housing for the staff, etc. But I started the process. Fast forward a few months, and the Men's home was in Hot Springs. That is the beginning of the story.

Without sharing all the story, just know that it was difficult. I had little help with running the program and I literally had to get married to get a day off. When we got back from our honeymoon, my wife and I lived in a house that was donated to the center. The only problem was that it needed plumbing work and the center didn't have the money to fix it. To complicate that, the center wasn't paying us. But things got worse. The house burned down with us in it.

Over the next few months, my wife and I lived as newlyweds in many different places until someone was nice enough to let us stay in their rental trailer for two and a half months. We still weren't getting paid regularly, which wasn't much anyway. To make matters worse, the city of

Hot Springs told us to get rid of the burnt house. The guys in the program and I tore down that house where we almost died.

Over the six months I was in Hot Springs, I looked at a number of properties for consideration for relocating the men's home. This was a step of faith since we had no money, but things finally came to a head. With little time off, not getting paid, being newlyweds, and a house fire, I was pushed to the brink. I finally said to the Lord, I want to go back to Little Rock. I gave up and the Lord let me. We closed the Hot Springs program down and moved the guys back to Little Rock. Eventually, I would go to another program. But you know where the Arkansas Teen Challenge is located today? In Hot Springs, Arkansas, at the very property at which I was looking. I gave up too soon. I didn't trust God to help me through the difficulty. He got someone else to get the program to Hot Springs. I'm not beating myself up but using it as a learning experience. At 24 years old, I was a newlywed with no business background and little help, but like Abraham, I should have stayed put (Promised Land was Hot Springs) and allowed the Lord to help me through the problem. Let me share the second story with you.

Bob leaves the Promised Land the second time

Not long after returning to Little Rock, the Lord led me to another program associated with Teen Challenge of Arkansas. When we went to the program, it was totally shut down because the director resigned and the boys were sent to my program in Little Rock. We worked there for two and a half years and turned the program around. God led staff to us, helped me raise support, and got us in the black. I was ready to spend the rest of my life there. Then the board asked me to resign. I was shocked. Here is what led up to that moment.

Six months before, I was walking down a dirt road next to the center and praying. About a half a mile from the center was a 100-year-old house with the windows busted out and generally ready to be torn down. At that moment, the Lord spoke to me, "Start a girls' home." This was not my imagination; a girls' home was the farthest thing from my mind. As always, I asked the Lord for confirmation. In the meantime, I told a board member, the one who lived locally and was instrumental in starting the original program, that I though the Lord wanted us to start a girls' home in that old house. He knew the owner and said, "No way. The house isn't worth it." That was the end of the story for him. Over the next 30 days some amazing things happened.

First, the owner of the old house lived about 200 miles away in Little Rock. He returned to the area for the first time in a long time and saw his old home with their gravesite beside the house and couldn't stand the way it looked. There was 200 acres of farmland with the house.

Second, a couple showed up at the center and said that they felt the Lord wanted them to be house parents for a girls' home. They were farmers and would have been able to take care of the land associated with the house. What is the chance of that happening?

Third, during that same month, the Lord called me to fly. Right next to the old farmhouse was a half-a-mile field that could have been used to fly me to the public relations and fund-raising meetings I was regularly holding. The program was in the middle of nowhere. The big town of about 1000 people was 13 miles away. Fayetteville, Arkansas was 35 miles way over winding roads.

Fourth, we got the house. The owner leased it to us for one dollar a month and put in new windows, siding, septic tank, as well as a new kitchen, bathroom, and bedrooms. And he was ready to spend more because there were four large bedrooms upstairs that could be used for girls.

Instead of using it for a girls' home, it became a staff house. One of the couples working for us moved into the house. The board wanted to move my wife and I into a living situation with another couple. When we first moved there, my wife, Dana, and I slept on a single bed in a small bedroom in the center for eight and a half months. We used a common bathroom but we made those sacrifices to keep the program alive until we could move to the house on the hill. The center owned 45-acres that had a house on it. The former director was still there trying to figure out where he was supposed to go.

Dana cooked for the boys in a commercial kitchen that needed new windows and a better source of heat. In the wintertime, hamburger meat wouldn't thaw out. In the summer, with no air conditioning in the kitchen and holes in the screens, we had to have fly-patrols to kill flies before meals. I'm not making this up. We would kill thousands of flies before each meal. It felt like we were living in a developing nation.

Eventually, Dana and I moved to the house on the hill where we lived for over a year and a half. The board sold the property against my objection and wanted to move us in the with the other couple and I told them

"No." I was believing for a place of our own away from the center. So, they fired me. I'm sure that they had their reasons.

Today, that program is doing very well but still doesn't have a girls' home. Though it is doing well, it isn't where it should be in my estimate after over 45 years. So, what is my point?

Out of all the things that God did to confirm His will in this story regarding a girls' home, God's Will didn't get done. There is always resistance to God's Will. But the thing that has shaped my life is what I could have done to change the situation. The board asking me to leave should not have been the end of the story. I should have challenged them to pray about this for 6 months before making a decision. But I didn't. It was so easy to leave and so hard to stay. They didn't treat us very well. By the way, when we left, God dropped a youth pastor job in my lap and took very good care of us. It was so easy compared to residential ministry because we didn't have to live with the kids.

If the board had approved me to stay during those 6 months, I would have asked this board member to mentor me rather than undermine me like he did. He could have told me where I needed work and helped me to grow as a leader. I certainly had a lot to learn.

So, here's my message to the church. If you in a tough position at your job or as a pastor, for example, hang in there. Don't give up. Pray for the people that are giving you the most trouble and then humbly approach them asking for them to help you do your job better. If you are the person that is in authority, like the board member I mentioned, try to help people grow in his or her job performance. Understand that people in the ministry are not in it for the money. People in regular jobs aren't either. They are trying to live their lives and make a difference with the talents and abilities they have. Try to work with them and mentor them and help them to fulfill their calling. Imagine what it would be like to work with you as your own boss. You'll find it isn't so easy. That leads me to my third story.

## Bob stays in the Promised Land

Fast forward over 30 years. By this time, I am approaching the end of my flying career. I wake up one morning and realize that if I am ever going to be a lead pastor, then I had better get going. Unfortunately, since I had never been a lead pastor and was old, 58 years old at the time, no one wanted to talk to me. That is except troubled churches. One church I tried out for didn't vote me in. This church had issues. I felt like saying to them, "Don't you know who I am?" It was like asking the ugliest girl to the prom and she says "no." I was stunned.

Later on, in the same area, the church that split off of the first church asked me to preach. Eventually, I would become their pastor. I didn't know what I was getting into. It was a difficult turnaround church, but my previous two failures that happened over 30 years before caused me to stick it out. I retired from that church after eleven years at age 70. Today it is still a small church, but it is healthy and growing.

I told you about those stories so that you understand that living by faith is tough. The devil is going to fight you and he works against you sometimes through the very people that should be helping you. You see it in the New Testament where Paul reproves various people for fighting among themselves. Churches split over the dumbest stuff so get ready for battle.

You may be asking, "How does this relate to my cancer?" Glad you asked. As you face the various procedures, diagnoses, doctor visits, and question and comments from people, it is important that you stay centered on Jesus. He is your source of life regardless of the what the diagnoses says. A friend of mine, retired from teaching at age 65. A few months after retiring, she was diagnosed with stage-four breast cancer and given six months to live. She said, "It isn't over until God says it's over." I'm all for doctors and use them a bunch, but they are not God. My friend died after 15 years at the age of 80. Her faith shined brightly in the face of cancer and she far outlived the doctors' prediction. Our faith should be in our creator who can change the story. Put your faith in Him.

## Faith is pushing back against the status quo

Let's talk a little bit about faith. Faith is always pushing back against what is the status quo. It wouldn't be faith if it didn't require change. Abraham needed a change in order to have food to eat. The status quo was "There is a famine and food is scarce." The logical solution was to go to a place that didn't have a famine, Egypt. The place of obedience is not always the logical place.

Faith is needed when we don't have enough of something or we need help in a particular area, or we don't know what to do. There will be a time in our lives when God's Word stands in opposition to what is taking place in our lives. We choose what we are going to believe and Who we are going to trust. This reminds me of the year 2020 when Covid hit New Jersey where I was pastoring. We were not allowed to have church by the State of New Jersey and the County in which we lived. The first month of the pandemic, our offerings for the church went to one third of normal, but the bills kept coming in. No one knew what was going to happen. People were dying by the thousands close to where we lived. People were scared to go anywhere.

We had just started a remodeling project. We pressed on with the project through the pandemic and everything worked out. Volunteers, staff, and construction workers kept showing up and we finished the project. We had to lean on the Lord when we didn't know what was going to happen. If you remember during the early stages of Covid it was okay to go to Walmart and the liquor store but it was too dangerous to go to church...at least in New Jersey.

I call choosing to believe "The Discipline of faith." Every day, there are plenty of opportunities to choose to believe that God is big enough to handle our problems. Abraham chose to doubt and ran from the problem of the famine and look what happened. Abraham was worried that Pharoah would kill him and take his good-looking wife, Sarah. So, he had her lie and say Abraham was her brother. It was only a little white lie because Sarah[26] was his half-sister (Gen. 20:12). Pharaoh took Sarah into his harem. Fortunately, God afflicted Pharaoh and he somehow realized that Sarah was Abraham's wife. Pharaoh scolded Abraham and sent him on his way with

---

[26] Sarai's name would later be changed to Sarah (Gen. 17:15). I will refer to her as Sarah.

the additional wealth to make up for any inconvenience. God still watched over Abraham even though he made a mistake. God doesn't expect us to be perfect either.

Abraham went to Egypt because the Nile River provided water even during a famine since it was fed from the snow in the mountains. Using irrigation, Egypt often had food when others struggled, making it the logical place to go. This is an important lesson for all of us to learn. Because a place or situation is difficult does not mean that we should leave it. That place could be the very place we need to learn and to grow. That place of difficulty may be the very place that God wants to show His power to meet our needs.

Abraham again lies about his wife to Abimelek (Gen. 20:2). This time God appears to Abimelek in a dream, "You are as good as dead because of the woman you have taken; she is a married woman" (Gen. 20:3). Abimelek took the hint and returned Sarah to Abraham. Abimelek chews out Abraham for his lie and asked Abraham "Why" he lied. Abraham's answer is important to consider.

> *Abraham replied, "I said to myself, 'There is surely no fear of God in this place, and they will kill me because of my wife.' ¹² Besides, she really is my sister, the daughter of my father though not of my mother; and she became my wife"*
> (Gen. 20:11-12).

Does this sound like a man of faith? Abraham is struggling to trust God to protect him and to provide for him among godless people. Notice that instead of praying, he says to himself, "There is surely no fear of God in this place, and they will kill me because of my wife." He didn't pray but talked to himself. It is okay to use your God-given reasoning ability, but God goes beyond our ability.

> *"For my thoughts are not your thoughts, neither are your ways my ways," declares the Lord. "As the heavens are higher than the earth, so are my ways higher than your ways and my thoughts than your thoughts"* (Isa. 55:6-8).

In the above Scripture, God is talking. He says His ways are higher than ours. It stands to reason that we as finite people cannot understand everything about an infinite God. He was trying to teach Abraham to trust Him during the famine.

There is another lesson to be learned by Abraham and us as well. God told Abraham that He would give him the Land of Canaan and that He would give him so many descendants that he couldn't count them. He didn't have the child of promise yet and getting killed by someone would certainly lower his chances of having children. Abraham should have believed what God said. Notice what Isaiah writes after the previous verses.

> *[10] As the rain and the snow come down from heaven,*
> *and do not return to it without watering the earth and making it bud and flourish, so that it yields seed for the sower and bread for the eater, [11] so is my word that goes out from my mouth:*
> *It will not return to me empty, but will accomplish what I desire and achieve the purpose for which I sent it* (Isa. 55:10-11).

Just like rain and snow water the earth so that plants grow, God's Word accomplishes what He sends it to do. He said that Abraham would be the Father of many Nations and that settles it. Abraham is still learning.

48

Abraham didn't trust God to provide food for him during a famine. Now he doesn't trust God to protect him among godless people.

We might ask the question ourselves, "Is God able to protect us in dangerous situations?" Certainly, we need to live our lives with wisdom and not needlessly place ourselves in harm's way, but sometimes we end up in uncomfortable situations. My oldest daughter was deployed to Afghanistan as an army chaplain and my other daughter is a police officer. Dangerous situations constantly arise. My daughters must trust God to protect them and so do I. Trusting God to protect your children is one of the great challenges of parenthood.

In 2020, we were challenged with the Corona virus. I lived in New Jersey close to ground zero, and we were not allowed to have church for a while. Then, we were allowed to meet in the parking lot. Finally, we could meet inside with restrictions. Covid attempted to scare us to not trust God. It showed weakness in our faith and unfortunately drove many out of church, never to return. We need to trust that God can protect us.

Ultimately, this life is not our final resting place. Heaven is our goal. Yes, we should protect ourselves by considering how we live and where we go, but we shouldn't live in fear of Covid or anything else. We need to live our lives trusting God in a land that doesn't fear God (the land of Covid).

Abraham said they lacked fear of God, but that should not keep him from trusting Him. In fact, the more difficult the situation, the more we need to trust God. Two Scriptures come to mind that illustrate the need to trust God in difficult situations. The Apostle Paul, who often faced opposition, wrote both passages. The first one demonstrates the mindset he had.

*[8] We do not want you to be uninformed, brothers and sisters, about the troubles we experienced in the province of Asia. We were under great pressure, far beyond our ability to endure, so that we despaired of life itself. [9] Indeed, we felt we had received the sentence of death. But this happened that we might not rely on ourselves but on God, who raises the dead. [10] He has delivered us from such a deadly peril, and he will deliver us again. On him we have set our hope that he will continue to deliver us, [11] as you help us by your prayers. Then many will give thanks on our behalf for the gracious favor granted us in answer to the prayers of many (2 Cor. 1:8-11).*

This passage of Scripture comforted me when I was given the diagnosis of multiple myeloma cancer. Here's why. Paul writes, "We were under great pressure, far beyond our ability to endure, so that we despaired of life itself." He wasn't worried if he would be able to pay the gas bill or if he might lose his job. He was worried about dying. He doesn't give us the details of what was happening, but he admits it was "beyond his ability to endure." He reached the end of his ability. That is an uncomfortable place to be, but it is where God wants us to be. That was where I was with my diagnosis.

Paul tells us why he was in that difficult position. Paul writes: "But this happened that we might not rely on ourselves but on God." We can't go wrong when we rely on God. That doesn't mean we don't do our best, but God helps us when we reach the end of our ability. That applies to sickness as well. We rely on God because at some point, modern medicine reaches the end of its ability. Our future is in God's hand.

Additionally, Paul writes about the future when he says that he has set his hope on God to continue to deliver him. My hope is in God for my future as well. He has everything under control.

It is important to notice that Paul went through the trial and God was with him. Living by faith does not mean that nothing ever goes wrong. It means that God walks with you through everything that happens in your life. That is what He has done with me as well.

The second Scripture is from Romans 4, where the Apostle Paul writes about Abraham,

> *[19] Without weakening in his faith, he faced the fact that his body was as good as dead—since he was about a hundred years old—and that Sarah's womb was also dead. [20] Yet he did not waver through unbelief regarding the promise of God, but was strengthened in his faith and gave glory to God, [21] being fully persuaded that God had power to do what he had promised* (Rom. 4:19-21).

This passage shows Abraham as a man of faith. We have already seen from the previous example that Abraham had faults and fears like all of us. He developed his faith through the trials and mistakes that he made. Seeing the imperfections in Abraham should encourage us to know that we too can grow in our faith relationship with the Lord. We will look more at Romans 4 in the next chapter.

### Ishmael

In Genesis 15, Abraham talks to the Lord during a vision. His concern was that his servant Eliezer would receive his inheritance since

Abraham had no child. The Lord confirmed to Abraham that he would have an heir.

This passage of Scripture presents a principle that all of us need to grasp; God gives us a promise and we should believe it. God told Abraham that his descendants would be as numerous as the stars. He believed God. Simple faith is so powerful. <u>Faith transforms the situation to conform with God's Word.</u>

Even after the promise of God in Genesis 15, Abraham was still having trouble believing that God was going to give him a child. In Genesis 16, Sarah is frustrated with having no children, so she offered her Egyptian slave Hagar with whom to have a child. This sounds foreign to us, but it was a common practice in that culture to have children through slaves. We see the same practice when Jacob has children through two of his wives' slaves. Ishmael would eventually be born and would be the source of problems between Hagar and Sarah. Eventually, Sarah would make Abraham send Hagar and Ishmael away.

It is essential to understand the statement: Faith transforms the situation to conform with God's Word. When God's Word says something, the situation may not look like the statement is correct. For example, God's Word says, "And my God will meet all your needs according to the riches of his glory in Christ Jesus" (Phil. 4:19). It may look hopeless, but God's Word is true.

Sometimes, however, people will quote this Scripture without considering the context of the statement. The Apostle Paul is speaking to the people of Philippi. Does this message apply to anyone and everyone? Notice what Paul wrote starting in verse 14.

> *¹⁴ Yet it was good of you to share in my troubles.*
> *¹⁵ Moreover, as you Philippians know, in the early days of your acquaintance with the gospel, when I set out from Macedonia, not one church shared with me in the matter of giving and receiving, except you only; ¹⁶ for even when I was in Thessalonica, you sent me aid more than once when I was in need.* (Phil. 4:14-16).

The Apostle Paul had a history with the Philippians. They were the only ones to give to him support when he first met them. He encourages them by writing that God would supply their needs because they had given. Often people try to glean the blessings of God without being obedient in giving.

Maybe your situation is desperate, and you have no money to pay your bills and no food in the house. Maybe you lost your job. Does God's Word still apply to you? Of course, it does. However, changing one's situation may require time. Not only may someone need to learn to give, but they may also need to learn to handle their money better. A person who begins tithing should expect, however, God to begin to work on their behalf.

Part of the change that needs to take place in each of us is our need for things. Notice how Paul addresses this issue.

> *¹⁰ I rejoiced greatly in the Lord that at last you renewed your concern for me. Indeed, you were concerned, but you had no opportunity to show it. ¹¹ I am not saying this because I am in need, for I have learned to be content whatever the circumstances. ¹² I know what it is to be in need, and I know what it is to have plenty. I have learned the secret of being content in*

*any and every situation, whether well fed or hungry,
whether living in plenty or in want. [13] I can do all this
through him who gives me strength* (Phil. 4:10-13).

There are a couple of powerful statements that the Apostle Paul makes. The Philippians were concerned for Paul and showed it through their giving. He makes a statement that he has learned to be content regardless of the situation. Contentment is a lesson that Americans need to learn. Our whole economy and advertising system is based on making you want something that you don't have: a bigger car, a newer car, a bigger house, a newer house, etc. We have a consumer-driven economy that expects us to buy stuff whether we need it or not.

Paul says he has learned the secret of being content. This is a difficult but necessary skill for us to develop. In fact, it requires help from the Almighty. Paul writes, "I can do all this through him who gives me strength" (Phil. 4:13). God gives him strength to be content. Certainly, God does empower us to accomplish many things, but the context of this verse is referring to Paul being content with his situation. God helps him with that challenge of having little and having an abundance. Obviously, the want for things is a challenge all of us face and we need help from God to control our desires.

Jesus has a great deal to say about possessions. It is a little bit scary. Jesus is approached by a rich young man who asked what he had to do to get eternal life. Jesus told him to keep the commandments, which the young man said he did. Then Jesus told him to sell his possessions, give to the poor, and come follow me. The young man went away sad because he had

54

great wealth and didn't want to part with it. But that is not the scary part. Look what Jesus said next.

> [23] *Then Jesus said to his disciples, "Truly I tell you, it is hard for someone who is rich to enter the kingdom of heaven.* [24] *Again I tell you, it is easier for a camel to go through the eye of a needle than for someone who is rich to enter the kingdom of God."* (Matt. 19:23-24).

Jesus' statement upset the disciples. They wanted to know who could possibly get to heaven then. There are a couple of reasons that the disciples are astonished by Jesus' answer. Craig Blomberg, a professor at Denver Seminary, writes,

> *The disciples respond in amazement, perhaps reflecting the Jewish tradition that equated riches with God's blessing. If those usually viewed as most blessed by God are so unlikely to make it into the kingdom, who in the world stands a chance (v. 25)? Jesus replies that, humanly speaking, no one does. But God can and does regenerate hearts, making it possible to serve him rather than mammon, which is otherwise everyone's "bottom line" (cf. 6:24).* [27]

The Prosperity Gospel preaches that believers are entitled to the blessings of Abraham and riches demonstrate the favor of God. Jesus, however, warns of the danger of riches in this passage and others. In the Sermon on the Mount Jesus says,

> [19] *"Do not store up for yourselves treasures on earth, where moths and vermin destroy, and where thieves break in and steal.* [20] *But store up for yourselves treasures*

---

[27] Craig Blomberg, *Matthew, The New American Commentary*, Vol. 22 (Nashville: Broadman & Holman Publishers, 1992), 300.

*in heaven, where moths and vermin do not destroy, and where thieves do not break in and steal. [21] For where your treasure is, there your heart will be also"* (Matt. 6:19-21).

Jesus warns about storing up treasures on earth because of the certainty of attaching one's heart to one's treasures. Additionally, wealth has the effect of covering up any spiritual needs with possessions that can hide the true condition of the heart. Just a few verses later, Jesus says, you can't serve two masters, God and money. Each of us must make a decision because it is not possible to serve both (Matt. 6:24).

Once a guy asked Jesus to make his brother divide the inheritance with him. Jesus warned him about greed and how life isn't measured by how much stuff you have. Then Jesus told a parable about a rich man that had a great harvest and decided he needed more storage space, so he decided to tear the old barns down and build new ones. The man then decided that he could relax and take things easy. God told the man that he was a fool because he was going to die and then whose wealth would it be. Jesus related that story to anyone that keeps things for themselves without a relationship with God (Luke 12:16-21).

With the Prosperity Gospel centered on the blessings of Abraham, it enters the danger zone, leaving its followers looking for their rights and wealth now with little thought towards eternity. Remember, our hearts go where our treasure is. This can be overcome by being aware of the danger and doing what Jesus said about putting God first (Matt. 6:33). Jesus helps us to center our lives, energy, and focus on the correct things if we let Him. The key is to be rich towards God.

Our sole purpose to study about faith is to help us live in a way that pleases the Father. Jesus talks about living for him when He talks about the cost of discipleship in the book of Luke. He compares loving Him to loving our family. He says we have to hate our families in comparison to loving Him. In that same passage, He talks about taking up our cross and following Him. He talks about counting the cost before you commit to serving Him. He compares it to a king going to war and deciding if he has enough resources to win the battle. He finishes this section saying, "In the same way, those of you who do not give up everything you have cannot be my disciples" (Luke 14:33). That certainly doesn't sound like the preaching of the Prosperity Gospel. Its focus is now.

# CHAPTER 4: ABRAHAM PART TWO

## Romans 4

I mentioned Romans 4 briefly a few pages back. Let's look at it more closely. The principles found in this chapter are life changing. To grasp the impact of this chapter, however, we need to remember the growth that took place in Abraham's faith. We have already mentioned some of Abraham's mistakes. Though Abraham is considered the father of faith, he had to grow into that position. His mistakes help us to know that we too can grow in our faith, faith that will help us through any situation. Romans chapter 4 gives us a view of Abraham after decades of growing in his faith. Let's examine what the passage teaches us.

> [18] *Against all hope, Abraham in hope believed and so became the father of many nations, just as it had been said to him, "So shall your offspring be."* [19] *Without weakening in his faith, he faced the fact that his body was as good as dead—since he was about a hundred years old—and that Sarah's womb was also dead.* [20] *Yet he did not waver through unbelief regarding the promise of God, but was strengthened in his faith and gave glory to God,* [21] *being fully persuaded that God had power to do what he had promised.* [22] *This is why "it was credited to him as righteousness"* (Rom. 4:18-22).

I have broken this Scripture down into five areas. Each one offers us helpful information required for us to live in faith in this world.

## Against All Hope

When you believe God's Word, there is always something that is going to contradict it. This happened to Abraham. It says, "Against all hope." There was nothing or no one in Abraham's life to give him hope that Sarah was going to have a child, except that God told him so years before. There weren't any medical professionals to tell him that they had something to help him have this child. Abraham and Sarah were both past child rearing age. Physically, they had no hope that they would ever have children. However, that is the point. When God does something, He wants us to know that He did it. It was beyond the realm of possibility for Abraham and Sarah to have a child...that is, except for the miracle working power of God.

As we live for God, we want to be open to God's miracles and go beyond what we can do alone. God can use us when we are obedient and look to Him for solutions. I am reminded of the story of King Hezekiah and his situation. This story is so important that it is found in three places in the Bible (2 Chron. 32:1-23; 2 Kings 18:17-19:37; Isa 36:1-37:38).

King Hezekiah brought about amazing spiritual reforms in his country of Judah. Despite the good that he did, the Bible tells us that the Assyrian King, Sennacherib, came against him. This brings up the point again that Hezekiah did everything right. He sought the Lord and reformed his country, but still the enemy came against him. Living obediently for God does not exempt you from the attacks of the enemy. It is during the attacks that God does amazing things. That is where each of us must depend on God to help us through.

The Assyrian king coming against Jerusalem was a big deal. He had defeated every king he came against. His army was known for terrible things that they did to the people they conquered. This was Hezekiah and his people's worst nightmare.

Sennacherib's armies positioned for attack outside the walls of Jerusalem. They attempted to get Hezekiah and his people to surrender by convincing them that their rebellion against Assyria would be unsuccessful. Hezekiah sent word to Isaiah the prophet and Isaiah prayed. God answered Isaiah's prayer by sending a rumor of another army approaching so Sennacherib withdrew to respond. As Sennacherib left, however, he sent a letter to King Hezekiah attempting to discourage Hezekiah from trusting in His God. In his letter, Sennacherib details the other nations and their gods that he had destroyed. He warns Hezekiah to not trust his god to protect him.

So here is the point. The first time, when Sennacherib's army was outside the wall of Jerusalem, Hezekiah sent word to Isaiah the prophet to have him pray to his God. God answered Isaiah's prayer and the Assyrian army left. Then Sennacherib sent his threatening letter. This time Hezekiah's response was different. This time he prayed.

*14 Hezekiah received the letter from the messengers and read it. Then he went up to the temple of the LORD and spread it out before the LORD. 15 And Hezekiah prayed to the LORD: 16 "LORD Almighty, the God of Israel, enthroned between the cherubim, you alone are God over all the kingdoms of the earth. You have made heaven and earth. 17 Give ear, LORD, and hear; open your eyes, LORD, and see; listen to all the words Sennacherib has sent to ridicule the living God.*

*<sup>18</sup> "It is true, LORD, that the Assyrian kings have laid waste all these peoples and their lands. <sup>19</sup> They have thrown their gods into the fire and destroyed them, for they were not gods but only wood and stone, fashioned by human hands. <sup>20</sup> Now, LORD our God, deliver us from his hand, so that all the kingdoms of the earth may know that you, LORD, are the only God"* (Isa. 37:14-20).

This time Hezekiah personally took the letter into the temple, spread it out before God on the altar, and prayed to God. It is one thing to get others to pray for your situation, but it is a different story when each of us learn to intercede to Almighty God for ourselves. God's Word tells us to boldly come before His throne when we have needs (Heb. 4:16).

You have an advantage over King Hezekiah. If you have accepted Jesus as your Lord and Savior, you have Jesus as your high priest interceding for you. God answered Hezekiah's prayer and destroyed the Assyrian army with a plague. When Sennacherib returned home, his own sons assassinated him. This is a story that shows what happens when you pray and trust God even when it looks like there is no hope.

Abraham's story became more public when God changed his name. Strassner writes,

> *In chapter 17, both Abram and Sarai had their names changed by God himself. Abram ("exalted father") became Abraham ("father of a multitude"). And Sarai became Sarah, which means "princess." Why did God change their names? As a symbol of their changed status! Abraham was now living under God's covenant blessings. And Sarah was now God's princess, destined to be the mother of Israel! They had gone from barren to blessed.*

*And, in the ancient context in which they lived, such a change called for brand new names.*[28]

When God had them change their names, people probably ridiculed them. There was no one encouraging them to believe in the impossible. It was a step of faith for them to change their name. When God gives you a promise, it is most likely against what the situation looks like. That is why you need faith.

Next, the author of Hebrews gives examples of people that had faith. He gives a general statement about faith that seems easy to grasp but is quite difficult. I wrote about this earlier in chapter two. The author of Hebrews writes we can't please God without faith which he defines as believing that God exists. Also, the author explains that God rewards those that earnestly seek him (Heb. 11:6). We need to renew our minds to fully grasp God's Word. Abraham renewed his mind and because of that was able to grasp God's promise of having enough descendants to create many nations (Rom. 4:18).

The Apostle Paul writes about the battle we have in our minds.

*[3] For though we live in the world, we do not wage war as the world does. [4] The weapons we fight with are not the weapons of the world. On the contrary, they have divine power to demolish strongholds. [5] We demolish arguments and every pretension that sets itself up against the knowledge of God, and we take captive every thought to make it obedient to Christ (2 Cor. 10:3-5).*

---

[28] Kurt Strassner, *Opening up Genesis*, (Leominster, England: Day One Publications, 2009), 77.

The Apostle Paul recognizes that we live in this world, but the way we operate is different once you ask Jesus into your heart. We wage warfare differently. The weapons we use are God's weapons and have the divine power to overcome the enemy's strongholds.

Paul also mentions another key place of conflict where we must have victory: our minds. He writes of demolishing arguments and pretenses that set themselves against the knowledge of God. That is exactly what happens. The Word of God stands in opposition to a world system. We must not allow our minds to go the wrong directions. The way we do that is through study and meditation on God's Word.

Christian meditation is different than eastern meditation. Richard Foster, one of the leading authors on discipleship, writes,

> *Eastern meditation is an attempt to empty the mind; Christian meditation is an attempt to fill the mind. The two ideas are quite different.*
>
> *Eastern forms of meditation stress the need to become detached from the world. There is an emphasis upon losing personhood and individuality and merging with the Cosmic Mind....There is no God to be attached to or to hear from. Detachment is the final goal of Eastern religion.*[29]

Christian meditation is where you think about a passage of Scripture. You may repeat it many times thinking about how it applies to your life. During this process, the Holy Spirit can make you understand how

---

[29] Richard J. Foster, *Celebration of Discipline: The Path to Spiritual Growth* (New York: HarperOne 1998), 20-21.

the passage of Scripture affects your life. Simply said, meditation takes the Scripture from your head to your heart.

## Without Weakening in His Faith

Battles should not weaken your faith. They should strengthen your faith and give you more confidence. Let me give you an example. I enjoy watching NFL football. I don't understand it, but to me, it is fascinating on so many levels. During preseason last year, all the rookies were contending for a few spots on the roster and each team had to make massive cuts in personnel before the regular season started.

During one play, a rookie caught a pass. The pass was only a couple of yards, but the commentator explained the importance of what the catch meant. It was the rookie's first catch in the NFL and, as the commentator explained, increased his confidence. The catch demonstrated to the rookie that he could play at the elevated level of the NFL. With all the lights, cameras, fans screaming, the increased speed and size of the players, he was able to focus on the play and complete the pass before he got tackled and then held onto the ball. With each successful play, he will grow in his confidence and in his ability to compete in the NFL. Each successful catch is like a battle, and battles should make us stronger.

As we live for God, doing things that we know are pleasing to God gives us confidence. Of course, we need God's help to live for Him, but our will is involved, and temptation is constantly around us. When we accomplish the right thing, it is like a completed pass. It builds confidence in our ability, with God's help, to live for him.

Abraham must have felt like a failure each time he goofed up. Finally, God found him faithful and gave him a son when he was 100 years old. For 25 years he waited for the promise to be fulfilled. But then came the ultimate test recorded in Genesis 22.

> *Sometime later God tested Abraham. He said to him, "Abraham!"*
>
> *"Here I am," he replied.*
>
> *[2] Then God said, "Take your son, your only son, whom you love—Isaac—and go to the region of Moriah. Sacrifice him there as a burnt offering on a mountain I will show you."*
>
> *[3] Early the next morning Abraham got up and loaded his donkey. He took with him two of his servants and his son Isaac. When he had cut enough wood for the burnt offering, he set out for the place God had told him about. [4] On the third day Abraham looked up and saw the place in the distance. [5] He said to his servants, "Stay here with the donkey while I and the boy go over there. We will worship and then we will come back to you"* (Gen. 22:1-5).

There are so many questions that could be asked at this point. Did Abraham talk to his wife, Sarah, before he took off on this adventure? Of course not. Notice that the Bible says that God tested Abraham. Do you think that God tests us? Of course, He does, but why? In this example, God is going to tell us. But first, what was the test? Abraham is told to take his son and sacrifice him as a burnt offering in the region of Moriah, which is where hundreds of years later Solomon would build the temple. Imagine what was going through Abraham's mind, "I waited 25 years to have a son and now God wants me to sacrifice him." That could have been his response, but instead he obeyed. The author of Hebrews writes,

> *[17] By faith Abraham, when God tested him, offered Isaac as a sacrifice. He who had embraced the promises was about to sacrifice his one and only son, [18] even though God had said to him, "It is through Isaac that your offspring will be reckoned." [19] Abraham reasoned that God could even raise the dead, and so in a manner of speaking he did receive Isaac back from death* (Heb. 11:17-19).

Abraham reasoned that God could even raise his son from the dead if necessary to fulfill His promise. A relationship with the Lord allows us to trust God even when it is difficult to understand why something is happening in our lives. The best part of the story is still to come.

> *[6] Abraham took the wood for the burnt offering and placed it on his son Isaac, and he himself carried the fire and the knife. As the two of them went on together, [7] Isaac spoke up and said to his father Abraham, "Father?"*
>
> *"Yes, my son?" Abraham replied.*
>
> *"The fire and wood are here," Isaac said, "but where is the lamb for the burnt offering?"*
>
> *[8] Abraham answered, "God himself will provide the lamb for the burnt offering, my son." And the two of them went on together* (Gen. 22:6-8).

What was going through Abraham's mind? What was going through Isaac's mind? Implied in Abraham's answer to Isaac was a prophecy about God providing a lamb which certainly could refer to Jesus' sacrifice centuries later. Now for the real test.

*⁹ When they reached the place God had told him about, Abraham built an altar there and arranged the wood on it. He bound his son Isaac and laid him on the altar, on top of the wood. ¹⁰ Then he reached out his hand and took the knife to slay his son. ¹¹ But the angel of the LORD called out to him from heaven, "Abraham! Abraham!"*

*"Here I am," he replied.*

*¹² "Do not lay a hand on the boy," he said. "Do not do anything to him. Now I know that you fear God, because you have not withheld from me your son, your only son"*
(Gen. 22: 9-12).

Abraham bound his son. The Bible doesn't tell us how old Isaac was. Estimates go from around 13 to much older. He could have resisted, but he didn't. He was like Jesus who voluntarily gave His life for us. Abraham raised his knife into the air and was on the downswing when he was told to stop. The reason is instructive to us. "Now I know that you fear God." I like to add, "More than man," because of Abraham's tendency to be afraid of what man could do to him since he lied about his wife, twice.        That is the lesson for us. Do we trust and fear God more than we fear man? Do we trust God's ability to direct our lives even when we don't understand? Do we trust God to protect us in dangerous and uncomfortable situations? Do we trust God in the middle of sickness, including cancer? Abraham finally did. He became the man of faith that trusted God in all situations. It is liberating to trust God and place your life in His hands, regardless of the situation.

As the story continues, God would provide a ram for the offering. God would also reiterate his promise to Abraham because he obeyed.

Obedience is a big part of living by faith for God. Living by faith is not about getting your rights fulfilled and getting more stuff, but about doing what God wants you to do.

Let's talk about obedience a little bit more. Suppose you get sick. You confess your healing and continue to get worse. Finally, you go to the doctor. You may feel like a failure because you didn't have enough faith to trust God for your healing but gave up and went to the doctor.

It is important to understand that God has placed His image in humanity. Humanity has come up with powerful medicines and technologies that bring healing to the body. They are not of the devil. The devil wants you to feel defeated when you go to the doctor. It is as if you don't have enough faith. He'll say things like, "If you can't believe God for your healing then what can you believe for?" Condemnation. The devil is called the accuser of the brethren (Rev. 12:10). We see how he operates in the book of Job when he accuses Job of only serving God because of the protection God gives him (Job 1:9; 2:4). The devil is real and doesn't have your best interest at heart. A life of faith is one that trusts God through sickness and health and through good times and bad.

God uses doctors and medicine. I told my cancer doctor that he was fighting the works of the devil. I called him Rev. Doctor. The point is that God uses doctors and medicine. Do we sometimes become too reliant on medicine? Yes, we do. Often, we fail to pray about our situation, but immediately go to medicine rather than God. God needs to be our first choice.

What do we do when a situation arises that contradicts what God's Word says? For example, when you can't pay your bills and you have been tithing. Let me share part of my own story. My wife, Dana, and I worked for Teen Challenge, a Christian drug rehab program. Back in the 70s, Teen Challenge was a tough ministry. It was low paying (when you got paid) and we were understaffed and overworked.

Once we were married, we lived in a house that was donated to the center. The problem was that the plumbing was messed up and the center didn't have enough money to fix it. That's okay, because on our first month-aversary the house burned down. We got out but lost most of what little we had. Fortunately, someone let us stay in their trailer for a couple of months. We weren't getting paid because the center didn't have enough money.

Finally, we shut the program down and moved back to the headquarters. We lived in an over-garage apartment. We still weren't getting paid, had little money, and almost no food. Finally, my wife had enough. She prayed and told God that if He didn't provide for us, He was a liar. Unbeknownst to her, Dana's sister, who lived a couple hundred miles away, was having a food drive for us at her church. She showed up with a U-Haul trailer of food the next day after Dana prayed. As a funny note, Dana saw the trailer and thought they were moving in with us, but it was a trailer full of food. God answered her prayer. That is an example of going boldly before the throne of grace and getting help.

Too often the enemy pushes us around because we don't know who we are in Jesus. We need to get aggressive and attack the enemy with God's

Word. It is important that our first response to problems is to turn to God for help. Look how Jesus handled temptation.

> Then Jesus was led by the Spirit into the wilderness to be tempted by the devil. [2] After fasting forty days and forty nights, he was hungry. [3] The tempter came to him and said, "If you are the Son of God, tell these stones to become bread."
>
> [4] Jesus answered, "It is written: 'Man shall not live on bread alone, but on every word that comes from the mouth of God.'"
>
> [5] Then the devil took him to the holy city and had him stand on the highest point of the temple. [6] "If you are the Son of God," he said, "throw yourself down. For it is written:
>
> "'He will command his angels concerning you,
> and they will lift you up in their hands,
> so that you will not strike your foot against a stone.'"
>
> [7] Jesus answered him, "It is also written: 'Do not put the Lord your God to the test.'"
>
> [8] Again, the devil took him to a very high mountain and showed him all the kingdoms of the world and their splendor. [9] "All this I will give you," he said, "if you will bow down and worship me."
>
> [10] Jesus said to him, "Away from me, Satan! For it is written: 'Worship the Lord your God, and serve him only.'"
> [11] Then the devil left him, and angels came and attended him (Matt. 4:1-11).

Each temptation Jesus said, "It is written" and quoted the relevant Scripture. If Jesus aggressively fought the devil by quoting Scriptures, then it is important for us to study and memorize Scriptures so that we have the knowledge we need to fight the enemy. "Do your best to present yourself to God as one approved, a worker who does not need to be ashamed and who correctly handles the word of truth" (2 Tim. 2:15). Not only is it important for us to use Scripture to fight the enemy, but it is also important for us to correctly interpret it.

Another reason to learn Scripture is because of the power of Scripture. "For the word of God is alive and active. Sharper than any double-edged sword, it penetrates even to dividing soul and spirit, joints and marrow; it judges the thoughts and attitudes of the heart" (Heb. 4:12). The Bible, God's Word, is not just a book. It contains words of life. It has the ability to reveal things about us to us so that we can change.

The Word of God is a weapon and listed as part of the armor of God in Ephesians 6. The Apostle Paul writes, "Take the helmet of salvation and the sword of the Spirit, which is the word of God (Eph. 6:17).

The Word of God is our offensive weapon. Notice that the Apostle Paul writes that our struggle is not against flesh and blood, but against an evil hierarchy in the heavenly realms. We are powerless to fight against this enemy without the Word of God. Our fists, guns, or knives don't work. That is why we need God's Word. That is why I have so much Scripture in this book, because I know that Scripture transforms people. It is powerful and reveals things to us.

God has given us the ability to pray. God has helped me so many times because I simply said, "God help me." Many times, the solution is immediate. Sometimes I must continue dealing with the situation trusting that God will help me. When dealing with sickness, don't get discouraged when you feel your body getting sick. Instead, begin to confess the Word. I am healed by the stripes of Jesus (Isaiah 53:5; 1 Pet. 2:24). We will look more at healing later.

Obstacles should not weaken your faith; in fact, they should rile you up to stand on the Word. There is going to be a constant battle between what God says and what the world looks like or says. Let's look at reasons that someone might weaken in their faith.

*Reasons for weakening in faith.*

Delay in the Answer

People often weaken in their faith when there is a delay in the answer. The lag between the promise and the fulfillment of the promise is time. While waiting, faith is required. Questions might be asked:

- Is God going to fulfill the promise?
- Did I understand the promise?
- Is God big enough to answer the promise?
- Does He want to answer my prayer?

During the questioning time, faith is needed. Abraham didn't weaken in his faith" (Rom. 4:19), despite contradicting information, Abraham believed God. Remember that Abraham took years to develop his faith. He weakened and left the Promised Land twice (Gen.12;20). He weakened and gave into his wife's request to take Hagar as his wife (Gen. 16). However, he was full of faith when God commanded him to sacrifice his son (Gen. 22).

## Not God's Will

Another method of dealing with delay is the conclusion, "It must not be God's will." In essence, the lack of fulfillment in a timely fashion has brought the conclusion that it's not God's will. The person gives up on the promise. It might be true that it is not God's will, but it could also be a copout and the person didn't continue to pray. It is important that we strive to know God's will and to understand His Word. We as finite beings cannot possibly understand everything about an infinite God. But God wants to answer our prayers and fulfill His promises. Gloria Beech Jackson, a former Assemblies of God missionary, presents a comprehensive theology of suffering in her book, *Through the Fire*. Her profound understanding of suffering has come from her own personal experience and enlightenment through those experiences. She writes,

> *"...God never answers prayers that are out of harmony with His character and His purposes. When the disciples asked Jesus to call down fire from heaven on some individuals who resisted His teaching, He replied that they did not know what spirit was animating such thoughts. God does not answer vindictive prayers. He does not harm individuals or manipulate them to make life more satisfying for someone else. He does not disregard an individual's freedom of choice by forcing that person to do right or to act in a certain way in response to another's prayers."* [30]

---

[30] Gloria Beech Jackson, *Through the Fire: Suffering as an Integral Component of Christian Life and Ministry* (Springfield, MO: Life Publishers International, 2011), 33.

The problem with giving up and using the excuse "It isn't God's will" is that it injures our faith in God for a couple of reasons. It has a negative effect on our desire to pray. We can begin to think, "What's the use? He won't answer anyway." This causes us to doubt that God has our best interest at heart. That is why it is important to strive to know God's will as we wait on answers to prayer. It can also cause us to go through the motions of praying without expecting any results.

It is important to understand that the devil attempts to confuse us about God's will and doubt God's intentions. This is exactly the tactic that the devil uses in the Garden of Eden. Look at the conversation between the devil and Eve.

> Now the serpent was more crafty than any of the wild animals the LORD God had made. He said to the woman, "Did God really say, 'You must not eat from any tree in the garden'?"
>
> ² The woman said to the serpent, "We may eat fruit from the trees in the garden, ³ but God did say, 'You must not eat fruit from the tree that is in the middle of the garden, and you must not touch it, or you will die.' "
> ⁴ "You will not certainly die," the serpent said to the woman. ⁵ "For God knows that when you eat from it your eyes will be opened, and you will be like God, knowing good and evil."
> ⁶ When the woman saw that the fruit of the tree was good for food and pleasing to the eye, and also desirable for gaining wisdom, she took some and ate it. She also gave some to her husband, who was with her, and he ate it. ⁷ Then the eyes of both of them were opened, and they realized they were naked; so they sewed fig leaves together and made coverings for themselves (Gen. 3:2-7).

The serpent first caused doubt about what God said. This continues to be a tactic of the devil to try to confuse us. The Apostle Paul encourages us to study and to correctly interpret Scripture (2 Tim. 2:15). If God's Word can be correctly handled, it can be incorrectly handled. That is why it is so important for us to regularly study it.

Next, the serpent calls God a liar. "You will not certainly die." Finally, the serpent reveals to Eve why God isn't telling her the truth, "God knows that when you eat from it your eyes will be opened, and you will be like God, knowing good and evil" (Gen. 3: 5). The serpent is saying that God doesn't have your best interest at heart and is holding you back because He knows that you will be God just like Him. The devil still uses this tactic to damage our trust in God and present us with half-truths. Therefore, we need to study God's Word and determine what God's will is and then stand by it.

Conflicting Information

Someone can weaken in their faith when the promise says something, but the facts in front of you say something else. It is imperative that each of us understand what the promise that we are standing on really says, so that we are not standing on sand instead of rock. We will talk more about this when we look at "Abraham facing the fact." One of the issues we face is that an infinite God cannot be understood fully by finite people. We can only understand what God wants us to understand about Himself. Study of the Word of God instructs us about the nature of God, His views on morality, human nature, and His dealings with humanity, but there is still much that we will not know about God until we get to heaven.

The prophet Habakkuk had trouble understanding God's ways. He complained to God about the sinfulness of the Jewish people and wondered what God was going to do about it. God tells him that He is going to send the Babylonians to deal with His people. This blows Habakkuk away. He couldn't understand how a Holy God could use the unholy Babylonians to discipline His people (Hab. 1:13). Habakkuk waits for God's reply. He thinks that he has stumped the Lord.

> *² Then the LORD replied:*
> *"Write down the revelation and make it plain on tablets so that a herald may run with it. ³ For the revelation awaits an appointed time; it speaks of the end and will not prove false. Though it linger, wait for it; it will certainly come and will not delay. ⁴ "See, the enemy is puffed up; his desires are not upright— but the righteous person will live by his faithfulness* (Hab. 2:2-4).

The Lord tells Habakkuk that the response that He is going to give Habakkuk is so important that he needs to write it down. During that time, writing material was expensive and difficult to use, but the Lord is emphasizing the importance of the message. Because the message was for others as well, the Lord instructs Habakkuk to write it plain enough so that the message can be delivered by a herald. Now for the message.

The message is for an appointed time, not then. "The righteous person will live by his faithfulness" (Hab. 2:4). The ESV and KJV translate it, "But the just shall live by his faith."

I can see Habakkuk scratching his head wondering what God meant. This message from God is so important that it is quoted in three other places in the Bible: Rom. 1:17, Gal. 3:11, and Heb. 10:38. We need to understand what it means. At the end of the book, Habakkuk finally understands faith. He writes,

> *17 Though the fig tree does not bud and there are no grapes on the vines, though the olive crop fails and the fields produce no food, though there are no sheep in the pen and no cattle in the stalls, 18 yet I will rejoice in the LORD, I will be joyful in God my Savior* (Hab. 3:17-18).

This is true faith in God. When everything doesn't go as expected, anticipated, or wanted, the faith-filled believer still trusts in God. As stated before, there is no way that a finite person can understand everything about an infinite God. There must be room in our theology for things that we don't understand. Habakkuk couldn't understand why God would use the Babylonians to discipline His chosen people. In the end, however, he trusted God's wisdom even though he didn't understand.

One of the problems with the Prosperity Gospel is that it is preached as a formula that always results in the desired outcome. As we saw in Hebrews 11, many went to their graves without seeing the desired result. The book of Acts is full of examples of struggle and difficulty. Steven was stoned, James was killed, and Paul was beaten and shipwrecked many times. The early church was littered with trouble and persecution. It would be nice if all they had to do was confess it away, but it was a battle. A spiritual battle was raging in the heavens. The problem with the American church is that it has been deceived into wanting heaven now.

I do believe that God wants to bless us, but the church must not focus on the temporal but the eternal. In an effort to convince people to live for God, the gospel message has been cheapened and many have sold people on the idea of blessings rather than obedience, victory rather than valor, comfort rather than commitment, and earthly rather than eternal. The Greek word translated "witness" is the word "martyr." The early church knew that to live for God could mean you gave your life, literally. Even today, many are martyred for their faith. In Revelation, John describes a great multitude that died for their faith. "And he said, 'These are they who have come out of the great tribulation; they have washed their robes and made them white in the blood of the Lamb'" (Rev. 7:14b). These are people that will give their life in the future.

Becoming a martyr is not something that anyone looks forwards to, but church history contains many that gave their lives. The enemy of our soul is always looking to cause trouble. Jesus said referring to the devil, "The thief comes only to steal and kill and destroy; I have come that they may have life and have it to the full" (John 10:10). This passage of Scripture presents the balance that is needed in the faith walk. God wants to bless us in this lifetime, but there will be battles. How we do in those battles revolves around our reliance on God and our knowledge of the Word of God.

Here are a few Scriptures that should be considered during our quest for the blessing of God.

> *6 But godliness with contentment is great gain. 7 For we brought nothing into the world, and we can take nothing out of it. 8 But if we have food and clothing, we will be content with that. 9 Those who want to get rich fall into*

*temptation and a trap and into many foolish and harmful desires that plunge people into ruin and destruction. [10] For the love of money is a root of all kinds of evil. Some people, eager for money, have wandered from the faith and pierced themselves with many griefs* (1 Tim. 6:6-10).

This passage of Scripture ought to make a person think about their life and where it is headed. Godliness with contentment is great gain. We are taught in America to want and not be content. But the apostle Paul goes a step farther. He says that those who want to get rich fall into temptation and a trap. The quest for riches is not getting you closer to God. What worries me about the Prosperity Gospel is that it focuses on what one can get out of the relationship with God.

I have preached that if you tithe, God will bless you. God has proved that to me. His Word says that He will bless you, but to make that your main focus is to invite danger. Paul continues saying, "Those who want to get rich fall into... foolish and harmful desires that plunge people into ruin and destruction." I am reminded of the Jim and Tammy Bakker story that covered the news for months. They started and ran the PTL (Praise the Lord) ministry for over ten years and developed an empire that included world-wide TV ministries and Heritage USA, a 2300-acre Christian theme park and hotel. The good that they did was overshadowed by the sex-scandal and the misuse of funds that sent Jim Bakker to prison.

What started out as a humble and powerful ministry got sidetracked into a lust for stuff. Paul calls the "love of money" the root of all kinds of evil and it sure showed in the Bakker story. Paul even goes so far as to say that people wandered from the faith searching for money. That is scary.

Jesus has a great deal to say about money.

> *²³ Then Jesus said to his disciples, "Truly I tell you, it is hard for someone who is rich to enter the kingdom of heaven. ²⁴ Again I tell you, it is easier for a camel to go through the eye of a needle than for someone who is rich to enter the kingdom of God"*
> *(Matt. 19:23-24).*

If we really look at Jesus' words, it should give us great concern about our view on wealth. We have so much in this country. Running water is wealth. Air conditioning and heat are examples of wealth. A car is wealth. A refrigerator is wealth. A cell phone is wealth. The list goes on and on. We have so much, and we need to examine ourselves to see where our heart is. Once again, Jesus tells us that our heart follows our treasure (Matt. 6:19-21).

Whether we like it or not, whether we want to or not, whether we believe it or not, our heart goes with our treasure. We can't help it. That's why Jesus warns us to not store treasures here on earth. You don't have to be wealthy to have treasures on Earth. Treasures are things that you value more than God. Paul called the "love of money" as a problem. Not having money but loving it. You can be dirt poor and love money.

Jesus tells us how to fix the problem. He tells us to not worry about things, but to seeking after Him first (Matt. 6:33). What will be given to you? You daily needs. But first, seek God's kingdom and His righteousness. It is all about our relationship with God and putting God first in our lives. Don't be obsessed about money but seek God first. Don't worry about the bills but seek God first. This is counter-cultural but will change your life if you do what Jesus said.

Let's continue looking at the life of Abraham.

## CHAPTER 5: ABRAHAM PART THREE

### Facing the Fact

The more I read this passage about Abraham, the more impressed I am with the strength in his life. Notice that it says that "without weakening in his faith, he faced the fact" (Rom. 4:19). Abraham was faced with a situation that was contradictory to what God told him, but Abraham didn't weaken in his faith. The lesson here is that contradictory situations should not affect our faith because we are rock solid in trusting what God has told us.

Not only did Abraham not weaken in his faith, he looked directly at his situation. Living by faith is not hiding your head in the sand but looking directly at the challenge. When I was diagnosed with cancer, I had to face the fact that I had cancer. I couldn't ignore it or confess it away. It wasn't mind over matter; it was trusting God to walk me though the battle. Abraham faced the fact that his body was as good as dead. But that is not the end of the story. Facing the fact helps you quantify the faith that you need. It gives you direction to search God's Word for His answer. It also helps you know that God must come on the scene because the situation is beyond you. You must trust God.

The Apostle Paul admits that he faced a situation that was beyond his ability to endure. He was worried about dying. He concluded that the difficulty he was in had a purpose: to help him not rely on himself but on God. Living by faith is relying on God. Here again is that passage in 2 Corinthians.

*⁸ We do not want you to be uninformed, brothers and sisters, about the troubles we experienced in the province of Asia. We were under great pressure, far beyond our ability to endure, so that we despaired of life itself. ⁹ Indeed, we felt we had received the sentence of death. But this happened that <u>we might not rely on ourselves but on God</u>, who raises the dead. ¹⁰ He has delivered us from such a deadly peril, and he will deliver us again. On him we have set our hope that he will continue to deliver us, ¹¹ as you help us by your prayers. Then many will give thanks on our behalf for the gracious favor granted us in answer to the prayers of many* (2 Cor. 1:8-11).

Let's talk a little bit about healing and medicine. The Bible tells us that God has placed in man His image. God's image inside of man has allowed humanity to be able to innovate, to create new drugs, have compassion on diseases, etc. That's the image of God producing good inside of man. Men and women still have a "sin" nature and need Jesus to be forgiven of their sins, but the good that we see inside of man is the image of God.

In the New Testament, Jesus is always healing people of diseases so I think that we can agree that disease is not a good thing, but of our enemy, the devil. Yes, sometimes God can get good out of a bad situation, like cancer, but I have a hard time believing that God's will is for someone to get cancer.

Assuming disease, including cancer, is of the devil, we can know it is God's will for us to fight cancer through prayer and medicine. Whatever the disease or ailment, and whatever the medicine, it still takes the God of creation and the human body working properly together with the "cure" to produce any results. Prayer, an attitude of trust in God, and confession of

His Word puts you in the best place for the best results. More of God brings healing.

It is okay to go to the doctor to get help. Take the medicine and believe God for healing. There is a limit to doctors and medicine, and when they reach their limit of their ability, then your only choice is to trust God.

Many believe that healing is included in salvation. If that is true, why are so many Christians sick? Is it lack of faith or lack of understanding of the Word of God? Many missionaries and great people of faith come down with cancers or other health issues that take them off the missionary field. What about Mark Buntain, dying in Calcutta and leaving his ministry in his wife's hands?[31] It was unexpected and unexplainable. Was that lack of faith or the attack of the enemy or God's will somehow?

These are very challenging questions. I do believe that we live below where God wants us to live and that we allow the enemy to beat us up when we should be victorious. Having said that, however, as I said before, there must be room in our theology for things that we can't explain. For example, what happens when we pray for someone to be healed and they die? Do we give up our faith? No. Do we walk around feeling defeated because we didn't have enough faith? No. We must trust the results to Almighty God. Whatever our situation is, we face it head on, believing that God has everything under control.

---

[31] Mark Buntain (1923-1989) was an Assemblies of God missionary who served in Calcutta, India. He is best known for his hospital and feeding programs serving some of the poorest people in the world.

## Did not waver through unbelief

As we continue looking at the life of Abraham, we will see a life-trait that sustained him through the difficult times. Let's look at what the Scripture says and then examine how Abraham got there.

> [20] Yet _he did not waver through unbelief_ regarding the promise of God but was strengthened in his faith and gave glory to God, [21] being fully persuaded that God had power to do what he had promised (Rom. 4:20-21).

There are some key points to consider:

- Abraham didn't waver through unbelief but was somehow strengthened in his faith.
- He gave glory to God.
- He was fully persuaded that God had the power to do what He promised to do.

Wavering in one's faith is easy to do. As a believer, you may have times in your life that you have trouble trusting God. The key is to not let yourself stay there but to grow through the difficult situation and continue to trust God and deal with the doubt and unbelief in our lives.

## Doubt

Let's examine the difference between doubt and unbelief. They are two different things. The word translated "waver" is also the same word translated "doubt." It is "diakrino" in the Greek language. "Dia" is a preposition that means "through." "Krino" means to judge. So, you are in essence judging through something. If you are buying a car, it is probably okay to "diakrino" the car. You are going to look at the engine to see if anything leaks and any fluids dripping. You want to listen to the sound of the motor and drive the car, etc. You are "judging through" the car to see if you want to buy it. You are taking in all the facts.

When you are dealing with what God says, however, it is not good to "judge through" what God has said because there is no way that you can have all the facts. Think about Abraham's situation. God says, "Go." He didn't tell him where, just "Go." Imagine if Abraham started analyzing things. "Well, God all my family is here. My wife's family is here. Our friends are here. My job is here, I have a home here." Abraham could have come up with a thousand reason to not obey God if he had tried to figure it out. But he obeyed. That is what God is looking for: obedience.

The problem is that when we are examining all sides of what God is saying to us and trying to figure it out how it can possibly be, we run into problems. When we take God's promises and turn them around and upside down and try to figure out things rather than accepting God at His Word, we end up not believing. God wants people that will accept Him at his Word. His ways are higher than our ways and his thought are higher than our thoughts (Isaiah 55:8). There is no way that we can possibly know all the resources that are available to God to help us or fulfill His promise to us. We need to believe and not doubt.

Let me share a couple of stories from the Bible that illustrate God's resources in two different ways. The first is found in 2 Kings 6. The prophet Elisha warned the king of Israel numerous times and helped him avoid conflict with the king of Aram. Once the king of Aram learned that it was Elisha that was revealing his military plans, he went after him. The king of Aram surrounded Dothan, Elisha's town, with thousands of soldiers.

When Elisha's servant woke up the next morning and looked outside and saw the soldiers, he was stunned. He asked Elisha what they were going to do. His response gives us a view into the supernatural power that God has available to us.

> [16] *"Don't be afraid," the prophet answered.*
> *"Those who are with us are more than those who are*
> *with them."*
>
> [17] *And Elisha prayed, "Open his eyes, LORD, so*
> *that he may see." Then the LORD opened the servant's*
> *eyes, and he looked and saw the hills full of horses and*
> *chariots of fire all around Elisha* (2 Kings 6:16-17).

Elisha saw beyond the physical into the spiritual. Though we may not have the privilege of seeing angels, we should recognize that the physical that we see is not our only resource. God is doing things behind the scenes in the spiritual realm and has many resources about which we know nothing. We need to trust that God can use those resources to fulfill His promises to us.

In the second story, God intervenes in another military situation. Samaria, the capital of Israel, is besieged by Ben-Hadad, king of Aram. People are starving and it has got so bad that people are eating their own children. The king of Israel blames Elisha and his god and plans to kill him. Elisha hears from the Lord.

> *Elisha replied, "Hear the word of the LORD. This*
> *is what the LORD says: About this time tomorrow, a seah*
> *of the finest flour will sell for a shekel and two seahs of*
> *barley for a shekel at the gate of Samaria."*

*² The officer on whose arm the king was leaning
said to the man of God, "Look, even if the LORD should
open the floodgates of the heavens, could this happen?"*

*"You will see it with your own eyes," answered
Elisha, "but you will not eat any of it!"* (2 Kings 7:1-4).

What an amazing prophecy! Elisha predicted an end to the siege, the
famine, and having cheap food within one day. The king's officer didn't
believe that even God could do that. Elisha prophesied that he would see it
but not benefit from it. God then sends a sound of horses, chariots, and an
army approaching to the Arameans, and they run for their lives leaving
behind everything, including supplies, horses, tents, clothing, weapons, and
money. When news reaches Samaria of the sudden withdrawal of the
Arameans, the people trample the king's officer to death running to pillage
the Arameans' camp. My point? God can meet our needs and keep His
promises regardless of how it looks.

## Unbelief

The second word is "unbelief." Unbelief is a wicked word. It is
"Apistis" in the Greek language. "Pistis" means faith. When you put the
"A" in front of it, it means against faith. Doubt is bad enough. It tries to
figure out God's promises rather than accepting them. Unbelief is much
more destructive. It stands against faith, against what God's Word says.

A good illustration of unbelief is found in Numbers 13. The twelve
spies have returned from looking over the land of Canaan. The Promised
Land was just like God said it would be, a land flowing with milk and honey.
The spies even brought back proof that God had told them the truth about

88

the land, but… We must be careful when we put a "but" in front of God's Word. The "but" for 10 of the spies was that there were giants in the land. There are always giants in the land. Giants are those things that are beyond you, that you can't control, that required God's help. If there weren't giants, then you wouldn't need God. You could handle everything yourself.

It is one thing to doubt, but unbelief takes it to a new level. Unbelief is like a cancer. It is contagious, and it will spread through the whole body. The ten spies were not satisfied to doubt God and not go to the Promised Land. They spread their unbelief to everyone that would listen. They got the people worked up until they were ready to kill Moses and choose a new leader to take them back to Egypt to become slaves again. God intervened by having the glory of the Lord appear and save Moses. Unbelief stands against faith in God. Unbelief questions the motives of God and sees Him as not having their best interests at heart. We need faith in God to trust Him at His Word.

Perseverance

Another consideration when talking about faith, doubt, and unbelief is perseverance. Perseverance provides the pillars that support the bridge of faith when things don't happen as fast as we think they should. Without it, we waver. Wavering is doubting. The book of James has a great deal to say about wavering.

*² Consider it pure joy, my brothers and sisters, whenever you face trials of many kinds, ³ because you know that the testing of your faith produces perseverance. ⁴ Let perseverance finish its work so that you may be mature and complete, not lacking anything. ⁵ If any of you lacks wisdom, you should ask God, who gives generously to all without finding fault, and it will be given to you. [6] But when you ask, you must believe and not doubt, because the one who doubts is like a wave of the sea, blown and tossed by the wind. [7] That person should not expect to receive anything from the Lord. [8] Such a person is double-minded and unstable in all they do* (James 1:2-8).

James writes about trials and the attitude we should have. If we understand the purpose of trials, it makes it easier to go through them. For example, when I do a workout that I haven't done in a while, I can count on having sore muscles. I may limp around for a few days, but I know what caused it and that good is coming from the workout. Spiritual battles can cause spiritual soreness, but they are developing perseverance in us.

Perseverance in the Greek language is "hupomone" and means steadfastness. But it means so much more. William Barclay, the late great University of Glasgow professor, explains it like this[32]:

> *Hupomone is not simply the ability to bear things: it is the ability to turn them to greatness and to glory. The thing which amazed the non-Christians in the centuries of Christian persecution was that the martyrs did not die grimly, they died singing.[33]*

---

[32] William Barclay taught at the University of Glasgow in Scotland for approximately 40 years. He was able to bring history, culture, and the Greek language into his teaching in such a way that it helped the student understand the significance of the verses.

[33] William Barclay, *The Letters of James and Peter* in *the New Daily Study Bible*, Revised Edition (Louisville, KY: Westminster John Knox Press, 1975), 49.

In another words, when we go through trials with the underlying strength that perseverance (Hupomone) provides, we walk tall with our shoulders back knowing that God has everything under control.

"Hupomone" is the ability to get up when one is knocked down. This is demonstrated in the movie *The Last Samurai*.[34] In the movie, Nathan Algren, an American Army officer played by Tom Cruise, was wounded and captured by samurai. As he recovers from his wounds, he learns the Samurai ways.

In one scene, Cruise ends up sparring with a samurai warrior using a wooden sword called a Bokuto. The samurai is soundly defeating Cruise, but each time Cruise is knocked down, he reaches out his hand for the Bokuto and gets up. The scene is filmed in heavy rain to make the dramatic effect even greater. You can't help but admire the image of perseverance that Cruise shows as he is unwilling to give up. That is the idea that James is trying to get across to us. Never give up.

The human spirit can do incredible things because God has placed His image inside of us. That reflection of our heavenly Father is what makes us creative, courageous, loving, determined, and able to accomplish amazing things. With God's help, we can stand strong in the middle of difficulty.

---

[34] *The Last Samurai*, directed by Edward Zwick, featuring Tom Cruise and Ken Watanabe (Warner Bros. Pictures, 2003), https://en.wikipedia.org/wiki/The_Last_Samurai.

Scholars often write about how the image of God was damaged after the fall of humanity recorded in Genesis 3. God Himself weighs in on this debate as He comments about the incredible ability of humanity in the Tower of Babel episode found in Genesis 11. The Lord has instructed humanity to go out and replenish the earth. In an act of rebellion, humanity has decided to stay and build a tower to Heaven. Here's what the Lord says:

> *⁵ But the LORD came down to see the city and the tower the people were building. ⁶ The LORD said, "If as one people speaking the same language they have begun to do this, then nothing they plan to do will be impossible for them. ⁷ Come, let us go down and confuse their language so they will not understand each other"* (Gen. 11:5-7).

The Lord says, "Nothing they plan to do will be impossible for them." Humanity has incredible abilities if it doesn't become discouraged and give up. At the time of this writing, my granddaughter is three years old. She has a tricycle but has not quite gotten the concept of peddling. If I push her on the tricycle, she can follow the pedals with her feet, but she doesn't push with her left foot. Before she has a chance to master the peddling, however, she is ready to do something else. Of course, she is only 3 years old, and I shouldn't expect too much out of her. This illustrates how our heavenly Father often views us. He can help us with our challenges (Pedaling a tricycle) for a while, but at some point, we need to learn to pedal for ourselves. We develop the perseverance when we keep trying to pedal.

As we live our lives in faith, God expects us to do our best and to persevere, but He will help us. We are waging war against the enemy: the devil. But we are fighting in an army led by the King of Kings and Lord of Lords. We are fighting in a war that we know that Jesus has already won.

Because we are in a battle, each of us must examine ourselves and see if we are allowing doubt and unbelief to undermine our relationship with God. Do we believe that He has the ability to help us live our daily lives? Do we believe He can help us pay our bills, manage our money, lose weight, heal our marriage, and bring about measurable change in our lives?

God doesn't expect us to be perfect, but He does expect us to grow in our relationship with Him. When you read the story of Joseph in the Bible, starting in Genesis 37, you are confronted with the development of a remarkable man. Joseph was spoiled as a child, but he didn't deserve the terrible life changes that happened to him. His brothers sold him as a slave, and he served 13 years as a prisoner until he was released and became the one of the greatest rags to riches story in history. He had to trust that somehow God was with him. The challenge for all of us to believe that God is somehow in control even when we can't see it. That includes being diagnosed with cancer or some other sickness.

Trials should help us grow in the Lord. Believers that never grow in the Lord do a great deal of damage to the church. First, they demonstrate that it is acceptable to not grow as a Christian, when the Bible clearly shows that is not acceptable. The Apostle Paul writes, "Therefore, if anyone is in Christ, the new creation has come: The old has gone, the new is here!" (2 Cor. 5:17). The old man is gone. The new is here. God is in the people-changing business.

Second, Christians that don't grow don't fulfill what God wants them to do in the body of Christ because they haven't grown in Christ. Paul also writes,

> Therefore, I urge you, brothers and sisters, in view of God's mercy, to offer your bodies as a <u>living sacrifice</u>, holy and pleasing to God—this is your true and proper worship. ² Do not conform to the pattern of this world, but be transformed by the <u>renewing of your mind</u>. Then you will be able to test and approve what God's will is—his good, pleasing and perfect will (Rom. 12:1-2).

Christians should present their lives to the Lord, including renewing their minds. That is the starting place. Next, Paul writes about the place that each of us have in the body of Christ.

> ³ For by the grace given me I say to every one of you: Do not think of yourself more highly than you ought, but rather think of yourself with sober judgment, in accordance with the faith God has distributed to each of you. ⁴ For just as each of us has one body with many members, and these members do not all have the same function, ⁵ so in Christ we, though many, form one body, and each member belongs to all the others. ⁶ We have different gifts, according to the grace given to each of us. If your gift is prophesying, then prophesy in accordance with your faith; ⁷ if it is serving, then serve; if it is teaching, then teach; ⁸ if it is to encourage, then give encouragement; if it is giving, then give generously; if it is to lead, do it diligently; if it is to show mercy, do it cheerfully (Rom. 12:3-8).

We must grow to fulfill God's role for us and not waver through unbelief.

## Fully Persuaded

Unbelief is based in fear. Unbelief is based in having a plan "B," or what you are going to do if God doesn't come through like you think He should. It is not all in with God. Being fully persuaded, however, doesn't come without effort. You must renew your mind. As we looked at the last page, Paul encourages us to renew our minds. He encourages us to not be like the world, but to be changed through a changed mind (Rom. 12:2).

Being fully persuaded involves offering your bodies to God as a living sacrifice. It has been said that the problem with a living sacrifice is that it keeps jumping off the altar. That is so true. We must offer our bodies daily as living sacrifices. We do that because of what Jesus has done for us. That is the least we can do.

Being fully persuaded requires us to surrender our will. It is not what I want but what God wants. The Apostle Paul writes,

> [20] *I have been crucified with Christ and I no longer live, but Christ lives in me. The life I now live in the body, I live by faith in the Son of God, who loved me and gave himself for me* (Gal. 2:20).

How should I be different when I am crucified with Christ? What does that mean? I have come up with a few ideas for me. You can make up your own list.

- My agenda is gone.
- My will is submitted.
- My anger is gone. Why do I get angry? Normally, I feel better about myself when I accomplish things that are on my agenda. But God's agenda may require me to do something different than what I have planned.

95

- Submitting my agenda to Him. This is how I crucify myself. Difficulties in completing my schedule due to interruptions may be the way that God is testing me.
- Allowing room for God to direct me.
- Drawing my personal worth from the value that God places on me, not from me accomplishing things, my position, or how much money I have.
- Each day I allow God to help me set my agenda.
- I fight temptations and don't allow sin to settle in my mind.

What does it look like for Christ to live in me?

- I am more loving.
- I am more aware of people's needs.
- I am more aware of the Spirit's leading.
- I am more willing to be used of God.

What does it mean to live by faith in the Son of God? Since I just quoted the Apostle Paul in the book of Galatians, let's look at more of his writing to better understand what he means. I'm using a passage from the book of Philippians. The church at Philippi knew the Apostle Paul very well. The story of Paul starting this church can be found in Acts 16. What makes this story so remarkable is that Paul and Silas ended up in jail. Despite being beat-up and bruised, they still sang praises to the Lord in jail. At midnight, an earthquake opened the prison doors and loosened their chains. What happens next wouldn't have happened if Paul and Silas had only thought about their agenda. They had plans and things that they wanted to accomplish, but jail time kept them accomplishing their goal of reaching so many people for Christ. But God worked despite their situation. Paul's agenda would have been starting a church in Philippi. But because Paul and Silas' suffering in jail, remarkable things happened.

After the earthquake, the guard, thinking that everyone escaped, was ready to take his own life, but Paul told him that they were all there. The guard was so moved by Paul and Silas' attitude in the midst of difficulty that he asked Paul, "What must I do to be saved?" The guard and his family would get saved that night because of the influence of Paul and Silas while in jail.

The influence that Christians have during personal adversity can be powerful. It shows the world around us that God is with us through trying times and that this life is not the ultimate goal. The congregation of Philippi grew out of Paul and Silas' time there, including their jail time. In his letter to Philippi, Paul explains his approach to life.

> [7] But whatever were gains to me I now consider loss for the sake of Christ. [8] What is more, I consider everything a loss because of the surpassing worth of knowing Christ Jesus my Lord, for whose sake I have lost all things. I consider them garbage, that I may gain Christ [9] and be found in him, not having a righteousness of my own that comes from the law, but that which is through faith in Christ—the righteousness that comes from God on the basis of faith. [10] I want to know Christ—yes, to know the power of his resurrection and participation in his sufferings, becoming like him in his death, [11] and so, somehow, attaining to the resurrection from the dead.
>
> [12] Not that I have already obtained all this, or have already arrived at my goal, but I press on to take hold of that for which Christ Jesus took hold of me. [13] Brothers and sisters, I do not consider myself yet to have taken hold of it. But one thing I do: Forgetting what is behind and straining toward what is ahead, [14] I press on toward the goal to win the prize for which God has called me heavenward in Christ Jesus (Phil. 3:7-14).

Paul's attitude is one of striving all out to have a relationship with Jesus. Everything that this world values, he considers worthless. His goal is to know Christ. This goes against much of what is taught in the Prosperity Gospel. The Prosperity Gospel focuses on a believer's rights and uses faith in God's Word as means to attain those rights. It is out of balance because it preaches little about obedience and what God wants. It is centered on getting wealth and what is yours because of your rights as a believer. David W. Jones is a professor of Christian ethics and director of the Th.M. program at Southeaster Baptist Theological Seminary in Wake Forest, North Carolina. He has also written about how the Prosperity Gospel has influenced the Gospel of Christ.[35] He writes,

> *Simply put, this "prosperity gospel" teaches that God wants believers to be physically healthy, materially wealthy, and personally happy. Listen to the words of Robert Tilton, one of its best-known spokesmen: "I believe that it is the will of God for all to prosper because I see it in the Word, not because it has worked mightily for someone else. I do not put my eyes on men, but on God who gives me the power to get wealth." Teachers of the prosperity gospel encourage their followers to pray for and even demand material flourishing from God.[36]*

As I researched who Robert Tilton was, it surprised me at the success of his ministry. He developed a church in the Dallas area called

---

[35] David W. Jones, *Health, Wealth & Happiness: How the Prosperity Gospel Overshadowed the Gospel of Christ?* (Grand Rapids, MI: Kregel, 2017).

[36] David W. Jones, "5 Errors of the Prosperity Gospel", The Gospel Coalition, June 5, 2015, https://www.thegospelcoalition.org/article/5-errors-of-the-prosperity-gospel/.

Word of Faith Family Church and at one time was the fastest growing church in America with a congregation of over 8000. His TV ministry reached around the world and he was known for preaching that Jesus wants you to be rich. He used his "Vow to God" donations that had to be made to his ministry.[37]

Tilton's website states,

> *"Because you are made in the likeness of a creative God ("in His image"), you will become very creative and find great wealth through that creativity. Jesus came here to teach us how to be abundantly supplied (John 10:10). As you begin to soak in this message, as you begin to hear with spiritual ears, God is going to begin to speak to you the same way that He has spoken to me in my life – and you will begin to have more and be more than you ever thought possible.[38]*

Tilton's ministry came crashing down as the media began investigating his claims of prosperity and healing, finding prayer requests in dumpsters outside his various locations. Today, he still has an Internet presence, but nothing like before.[39] Tilton represents the worst in the Prosperity Gospel message and messengers because it is all about money.

Money, power, luxury, and good health appeal to all of us, but you can see from the Apostle Paul's message that only knowing Jesus is his top

---

[37] https://en.wikipedia.org/wiki/Robert Tilton, Accessed March 25, 2023. This article details the investigation into his ministry and the many legal problems he has had.

[38] Robert Tilton Ministries, "How to be Rich and Have Everything You Always Wanted," accessed October 16, 2022, https://store.aegispremier.com/wof/product/Download/DWBK-01.

[39] "Robert Tilton", Wikipedia, accessed March 27, 2023, https://en.wikipedia.org/wiki/Robert_Tilton.

goal. I realize that everyone can't live like Paul because he wasn't married and had no children. Families always present challenges. Jesus puts life in perspective in His Sermon on the Mount. He tells us to not worry about this life, but to seek Him first. Jesus even contrasts how beautiful the flowers are and reminds us that they are even more beautiful than Solomon in all his glory. The birds don't prepare for winter but God takes care of them. He reminds us that worrying doesn't do any good and worrying is what the pagans do. He reproves us of having little faith (Matt. 6:25-33).

Jesus talks about seeking the kingdom of God first. Life isn't about the amount of stuff you have. Jesus tells us not to worry about what we should eat or drink or wear. His top priority is seeking the Kingdom of God or putting God first. For many people that could be a lifestyle change. How do you seek first the Kingdom of God? It is a matter of making knowing God the top priority in your life. Each of us need to carve out time to spend with the Lord, listening to His Spirit, meditating on Scripture, and studying His Word.

Seeking first should also bring about changes in our lives. We are told to not conform to the pattern of this world. What is the pattern of this world? The pattern of this world is "All about me and what I want", not what God wants. We observe the world view in TV commercials. They are all about you and me wanting something that we don't have. We are tempted to want stuff that is bigger, newer, prettier, faster, more expensive, and makes us younger. We feel good about ourselves because of what we drive, or where we live, how we look, or the clothes we wear, instead of what God thinks about us.

Renewing our mind helps us to think like God thinks and not like the world. It helps us to understand how God wants us to operate. It is counter cultural. To renew our minds, we need to not only read God's Word, but meditate on it. Christian meditation helps us to internalize God's Word and apply it to our lives.

As you meditate on God's Word, faith arises in your heart. Scripture tells us, "So then faith *cometh* by hearing, and hearing by the word of God" Rom. 10:17 (KJV 1900). The NIV says, "Consequently, faith comes from hearing the message, and the message is heard through the word about Christ" (Rom. 10:17). Faith is generated by hearing or understanding the Word of God and what God says about us. That comes through careful thought and meditation and illumination of the Holy Spirit. When we understand God's Word, it gives us something onto which to hold. Let me give you an example.

In the book of Psalms we read,

*1 Blessed is the man*
*That walketh not in the counsel of the ungodly,*
*Nor standeth in the way of sinners,*
*Nor sitteth in the seat of the scornful.*
*2 But his delight is in the law of the LORD;*
*And in his law doth he meditate day and night.*
*3 And he shall be like a tree planted by the*
*rivers of water,*
*That bringeth forth his fruit in his season;*
*His leaf also shall not wither;*
***And whatsoever he doeth shall prosper***
(Psalm 1:1–3 {KJV 1900})

This passage of Scripture starts off with "blessed." That means that you can see the favor of God on your life. Isn't that what all of us want? This is referring to more than financial fortune. We see many in our society and around the world that are financially wealthy and far from God. Blessing comes in so many other forms. I am blessed with two beautiful daughters, two wonderful sons-in-law and now two grandchildren. My wife and I have been married 47 years. She is my rock and encourager. Everyone is healthy. That is worth more than money. I am blessed. I have seen so many people that struggle because they violate the laws of God.

That highlights the next part of the passage. Who or what do you allow to influence your life? The "blessed person" doesn't walk in step with the wicked. It is important to be wary of those you associate with because they can influence you for evil. To prevent being influenced by the world, it is imperative for us to delight in the law of the Lord, the Bible. We are told to meditate on it day and night, not just to read a Scripture every now and then. It should be the center of our lives and will help guide us through the challenges that we face daily.

Foster considers study and meditation as part of the Spiritual Disciplines. He writes, "The purpose of the Spiritual Disciplines is the total transformation of the person. They aim at replacing old destructive habits of thought with new life-giving habits."[40] Foster further develops and differentiates the ideas of study and meditation.

*The process that occurs in study should be distinguished from meditation. Meditation is devotional;*

---

[40] Foster, 62.

*study is analytical. Meditation will relish a word; study will explicate it. Although meditation and study often overlap, they constitute two distinct experiences. Study provides a certain objective framework within which meditation can successfully function."[41]*

If we study and meditate on the "Law of the Lord" or the Ten Commandments, we can receive wonderful guidance for our lives. Notice Commandment number 10, for example, you shall not covet.

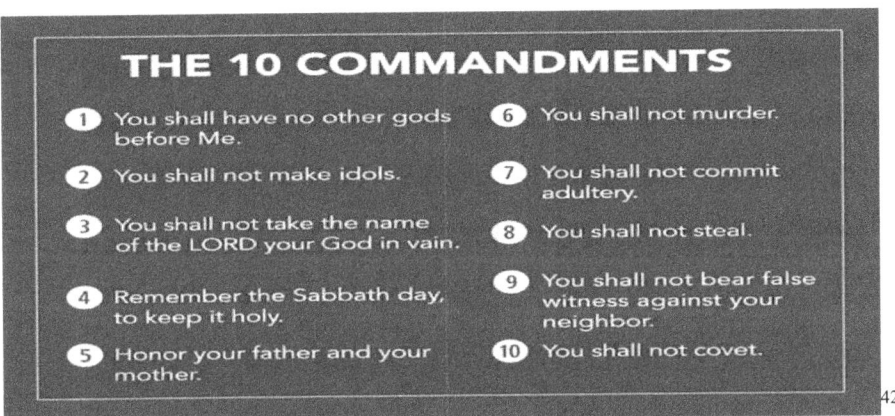

We are commanded not to covet anything including someone else's wife or animals. Our whole advertising system is based on making you want something that you don't have or coveting what someone else possesses. We want to dress with the best clothes and have makeup that makes us look like someone else, etc. As we meditate on Scripture, the Holy Spirit can show

[41] Ibid, 64.

[42] Mickey Elliott, "Understanding the 10 Commandments and their relevance for today," Reporter-Times, December 10, 2021, https://www.reporter-times.com/story/lifestyle/faith/2021/12/10/understanding-10-commandments-and-their-relevance-today/6457925001/.

us what we are coveting. The Holy Spirit can teach us where we need to change.

Look at commandment four, "Remember the Sabbath day, to keep it holy." Our society almost totally ignores this commandment. Because of that we see many industries operating seven days a week. I understand that some businesses must be open continuously, such as hospitals, but often that is not the case. Desire to make money can drive businesses to be open with no regard for God's law.

Many people work seven days a week. God did not design the human body to keep going without rest. We need rest to allow our bodies time to catch up and repair themselves. As we meditate and study this commandment, we learn how to apply it to our lives. It is also a step of faith to trust God that because He commands a Sabbath rest and we obey it, we will be able to get all the pressing stuff done with the remaining six days. I know that we live under grace, but the Ten Commandments were written for our benefit. All of them still provide guidance for our lives.

If we meditate on God's Word day and night and apply it to our lives, we will, according to Psalms 1, prosper in our way. That doesn't mean we won't have problems, but, generally, we will be headed the right direct. The rest of Psalms 1 contrasts a person that doesn't apply God's principles to their lives. They will have many problems that the person that applies God's principles to their lives doesn't have.

God expects us to believe His Word and then He works on our behalf. The best example of this is Abraham in Genesis 15. God tells Abraham that he is going to have a son as an heir. "Abram believed the

LORD, and he credited it to him as righteousness" (Gen. 15:6). Notice that believing what God says does not always fit into the possible realm. It was impossible for Abraham and Sarah to have a kid...except with God.

The Prosperity Gospel loses its way here because everything is about this life and possessions. Remember, Jesus warned us that we shouldn't store treasures here because our hearts become attached to them (Matt. 6:19-21). We as Christians must not lose focus on our eternal destiny. That being said, I do believe that God wants to bless us in this lifetime. Balance is the key to living our lives. Studying the Word of God and meditating on it allows the Holy Spirit the opportunity to correct when we get out of balance. We should also heed the warning that Jesus gives us regarding our heart being where our treasure is. If we value things in this life too much, it makes it more challenging for us to live all out for God.

As we live our lives, we are faced with situations that require us to make decisions. Sometimes our needs seem insurmountable. That is where we need God's help. It is important for us to include God in our daily challenges and ask Him for guidance. This requires faith. Do we believe that God can make a difference in our lives and answer our prayers?

The fact that we need faith means that there is going to be a time in our lives when we don't have enough of something. There will be a time in our lives when God's Word stands in opposition to what is taking place in our lives. There will be times when it seems like things are not going the way they should. This is when we must press into God's Word and build our relationship with the Lord. As Paul mentioned before, we present our bodies as living sacrifices.

Presenting our bodies to God includes everything we do. That means what we eat, our exercise, our sleep, etc. This is the vessel that God has given us and we need to take care of it and present it to God. But Paul tells us we need to renew our minds as well. How do we do that? First, we need to be careful what we put in our minds. Then, we need to replace the old with God's Word. What does God's Word say about a particular subject? That requires us to examine ourselves, not to put ourselves down but to learn what we need to change.

As a trumpet player, when I practiced, I listened to my playing and examined it, evaluating how it was and where change needed to take place. Also, I had to come up with a game plan for bringing about change. Change doesn't take place without planning and following through with the plan. That is where we need discipline. Let me explain.

If I want to improve my playing on trumpet, the first thing I have to do is get the trumpet out. That may seem like a simple and an obvious thing that must take place, but the first step is the hardest to do. When I want to exercise lifting the first weight or taking the first step in a run is the hardest to do. Why? Because our bodies don't want to do it. It is so much easier to sit on the couch and watch TV. Our bodies and our minds don't want to change. We must discipline them like a little child. Look what the Apostle Paul writes,

*24 Do you not know that in a race all the runners run, but only one gets the prize? Run in such a way as to get the prize. 25 Everyone who competes in the games goes into strict training. They do it to get a crown that will not last, but we do it to get a crown that will last forever. 26 Therefore I do not run like someone running*

*aimlessly; I do not fight like a boxer beating the air.*
*27 No, I strike a blow to my body and make it my slave so*
*that after I have preached to others, I myself will not be*
*disqualified for the prize* (1 Cor. 9:24-27).

Paul emphasizes the importance of discipline. Change doesn't magically happen. We must apply ourselves to change by adding discipline to our lives and making our bodies obey. Fasting is a good way to disrupt the control that the body has over us.

Fasting combined with meditation on Scripture is a powerful way to make changes in one's life. Meditation is a slow process and requires a commitment of time. A person reads over a passage of Scripture multiple times allowing the Holy Spirit to illuminate it to them. They ask questions and analyze how this passage of Scripture changes their lives.

Interpreting Scripture can be challenging. We must interpret it correctly. Our understanding of Scripture may challenge us to respond a certain way. When I was a new Christian in college, for example, I threw my contacts away and went without contacts or glasses for six months as "proof" of my faith in the healing of my eyes. My eyes never improved.

Faith has to be more than actions. It needs to be "fully persuaded", but that persuasion needs to be based in the proper understanding of God and His Word. Faith has to be more than a legalistic action. Often, we may think that we are having faith in God, but our faith is actually in our bank account, or our ability, someone else's ability or faith in our faith. God needs to be the basis of our faith.

Being fully persuaded means that we have battled with doubt and have defeated it. Doubt looks at something God says and turns it this way and that trying to figure it out. Faith that is fully persuaded takes what God says at face value. Being fully persuaded only comes through a relationship with God. As you get to know Him, you are able to trust your life to Him. Faith steps out when it can't see the results. Faith doesn't have to have all the answers. Faith trusts God when we don't understand.

As I have stated many times, there must be room in one's theology for the unexplainable. When things don't go as planned, we still need to trust in the Lord. Think about the Christians in the colosseum in Rome. Were they confessing, "The lion's not going to eat me, the lion's not going to eat me?" No. They were submitting their lives and the lives of their families to God. They were trusting God in that terrible situation. In their case, living for God meant giving their lives. Jackson deals with many questions regarding suffering including, "Why would God create a world where there would be so much suffering?" She writes,

> God chose, then, to create the world knowing it would become imperfect and broken—a world in which suffering would exist. So why did He do this? Because only in such a world could God exhibit His love in its highest and purest form, by His own voluntary death for the sake of the humans being He created and loved.[43]

Jackson further explains the benefits of our sinful world as the place where God's attributes could be revealed,

> Most importantly, only a broken, suffering world would provide a context in which God would have occasion to reveal the full depth of the most awesome

---

[43] Jackson, 6.

*core aspect of His being—love, which would allow the manifestation of His mercy and forgiveness.*[44]

As Jackson expounds on human suffering, she turns the equation around, looking at suffering from God's point of view. She writes,

*Therefore, the question is not, "Why does a good and loving God allow humans to suffer?" but, "Why does a good and loving God allow himself, the purest being, with the highest value in the universe, to suffer?" For God not to have created humans would have been to avoid His own inevitable suffering, since He knew in advance that, because of the perfect love inherent in His own being, He himself would suffer.*

*Therefore, when God chose to create humans, He chose in advance to suffer with and for us, the created beings whom He loved. He deemed that the ultimate end He would bring about—multitudes of His own children, purchased through His own pain and sacrifice, sharing His own nature and eternally delighting in His presence by their own free choice to belong to Him—had such high value to Him that He would allow, and himself endure, human suffering.*[45]

Jackson's understanding of suffering helps us understand God's motivation for it. Let me give a little bit of my own personal struggle. I retired as an airline pilot at the height of my career, four years early, to pastor a church. A year and a half after retiring, I was diagnosed with Multiple Myeloma cancer, for which there is no cure outside of God. I could

---

[44] Ibid.
[45] Ibid.

109

have asked, "Why Lord, after all I have given up to serve you?" I could have been bitter, but I trusted the Lord through the treatment.

I was placed on various drugs. Once the disease was under control, the doctors recommended that I have a stem cell transplant using my own stem cells. Before they could harvest my stem cells, I had to take various drugs and then have a port put in my aorta. The whole thing was a little scary and required me to trust the Lord. It didn't help when a young man that looked like he was in high school came into my room to talk with me about the port procedure. I assumed he was the aide and was emptying the trash. Then he told me he was the doctor. It was Doogie Howser, M.D. all over again. At some point, you may face a medical procedure that makes you uncomfortable. It is during these difficult times that we must trust the Lord.

One thing that I do like about the "Faith" or Prosperity Gospel is their stance on authority. Let me give a couple of examples. First, we, by faith, take authority over our situation in light of who Jesus is and who we are in Him. It is imperative that we understand that we are important to God and created in His image. Because of our importance, He sent His Son to die for our sins. Our relationship with Jesus allows us to boldly approach the throne of God for our needs as the author of Hebrews tell us (Heb. 4:14-16).

We have authority to approach the throne of God through Jesus. The problem is that if we don't believe that or know about it, then we won't use that authority. The "Faith" gospel taught me about authority.

Second, the "Faith" gospel taught me the importance of monitoring what I say. My words have authority. We will talk about this more in the following chapters.

# SECTION THREE: FAITH IN GOD

## CHAPTER 6: HAVE FAITH IN GOD

This passage of Scripture is an important for us to consider in our faith walk. Let's look at it in the context it is written. This is Jesus' final week before He is crucified. We need to carefully consider what Jesus is trying to teach us and His disciples.

> *[12] The next day as they were leaving Bethany, Jesus was hungry. [13] Seeing in the distance a fig tree in leaf, he went to find out if it had any fruit. When he reached it, he found nothing but leaves, because it was not the season for figs. [14] Then he said to the tree, "May no one ever eat fruit from you again." And his disciples heard him say it* (Mark 11:12-14).

The next thing that Jesus did was enter Jerusalem and drive out the money changers and those buying and selling stuff in the temple courts. This was the second time that Jesus cleared the temple courts. Jesus would spend all day in the Jerusalem and then leave the city.

> *[19] When evening came, Jesus and his disciples went out of the city.*

*20 In the morning, as they went along, they saw the fig tree withered from the roots. 21 Peter remembered and said to Jesus, "Rabbi, look! The fig tree you cursed has withered!"* (Mark 11: 19-21).

There are all kinds of explanations for why Jesus cursed the fig tree. Some say that it was because the fig tree had leaves and no fruit. He cursed it because it represented the hypocrisy of the religious leaders. James A. Brooks, a former professor at New Orleans Seminary and Greek scholar, writes,

> *The cursing of the fig tree and the expulsion of the merchants from the temple (11:15–19) are prophetic actions that symbolize the same thing, the coming judgment on unfaithful Israel by the destruction of Jerusalem and its temple. Israel, like the fig tree, appeared to be thriving; but the appearances were deceiving because Israel and the fig tree were bearing no fruit*[46]

To me, it appears that the simplest explanation is the best. I realize that often Jesus conceals meanings in parables from the average person and there are many prophecies that scholars still haven't figured out in the book of Revelation and other places in Scripture. However, we should ask ourselves the question, "Why did God give us His Word if it is too difficult to understand?" The answer is He didn't, but we must study it and the Spirit of God helps us to understand it. We read it in context and should be careful that we don't read something into it that God never intended. With that being

---

[46] James A. Brooks, *Mark, The New American Commentary, Vol. 23* (Nashville: Broadman & Holman Publishers, 1991), 180.

said, let's search for the simplest explanation for this passage as we examine the next few verses.

> [22] *"Have faith in God,"(Chapter 6) Jesus answered.*
> [23] *"Truly I tell you, if anyone says to this mountain (Chapter 7), 'Go, throw yourself into the sea,' and does not doubt in their heart (Chapter 8) but believes that what they say will happen(Chapter 9), it will be done for them (Chapter 10). [24] Therefore I tell you, whatever you ask for in prayer, believe that you have received it, and it will be yours. [25] And when you stand praying, if you hold anything against anyone, forgive them, so that your Father in heaven may forgive you your sins"* (Mark 11:22-25). (Chapter 11)

I have broken the passage down into chapters because there is so much to learn. In this chapter let's deal with "Have faith in God." The whole passage revolves around our understanding of these four words. I have listed some things it affects.

- When you have faith in God, it turns your whole perspective on life from this life to eternity. When we make decisions solely based on our earthly perspective, we lose sight of God's plan.
- Having faith in God makes us consider His will in our decision making. Every day we are faced with many opportunities to make timely decisions. We should allow God the opportunity to direct us.
- Having the attitude of faith in God allows us to be more open to the leading of the Holy Spirit as situations arise.
- Having faith in God allows us to see our situation, the world, and people differently. We become open to idea that God is orchestrating things in our lives.
- Having faith in God as the center of our attention helps us monitor our attitude and the way we respond to life. With God at the center of life, we should have a positive attitude.

It is more than positive motivation, but faith in God knowing He has our best interest at heart and is working on our behalf.
- Having faith in God should open us up to use our resources for God in new ways.
- Having faith in God is all about our relationship with the Father. It is front and center in everything we do and how we live.

Hebrews 11, the faith chapter, helps us better understand what faith is.

*Now faith is confidence in what we hope for and assurance about what we do not see. ² This is what the ancients were commended for.*
*³ By faith we understand that the universe was formed at God's command, so that what is seen was not made out of what was visible* (Heb. 11:1-3).

The NIV says, "Faith is confidence in what we hope for and assurance about what we do not see". KJV calls it "The substance of things hoped for, the evidence of things not seen." Faith is somehow knowing something that hasn't happened. That is forward-looking faith.

Faith can also be backward looking. Hebrews 11:3 says, "By faith we understand that the universe was formed at God's command." We weren't there, but we accept that God created the universe as fact by faith.

Both the backward-looking and forward-looking faith depend on having faith in God. They depend on our relationship with God. If we lack the relationship with God and the direction He gives us, then the next part we are going to talk about becomes little more than positive motivation.

There is power in having a positive attitude. I've read many sales books that speak of having a positive attitude. They tell you to put a picture on the refrigerator of the number of widgets you want to sell next month.

Immerse your mind in the goal that you have set for yourself. There is definitely power in having a positive mental attitude, and that includes speaking verbally what you intend to do. For example, I am going to lose 10 pounds this month. As a way to help me achieve my goal, I tell everybody in my family and at work, and anyone else that will listen. The power comes from having accountability and from keeping your goal at the front of your mind. Keeping your goal constantly in front of you and speaking it will hopefully help you do the things that are needed to accomplish your goal.

Positive motivation works, but it is limited in what it can accomplished. Our willpower doesn't have power to help us make deep changes in our lives. What we are talking about today goes beyond what can humanly be accomplished. Paul writes, "Therefore, if anyone is in Christ, the new creation has come: The old has gone, the new is here!" (2 Cor. 5:17). In Christ is a relationship with Almighty God that can affect change in our lives.

- Being in Christ can help us overcome addictions.
- Being in Christ can help us overcome deep-seated issues in our lives.
- Being in Christ can help us forgive those that have hurt us.
- Being in Christ can help us discover things about ourselves that we didn't know before.
- Being in Christ can help us in our marriage, help us raise our kids, and find our career. It is the way that we live our life as a foreigner in this world,

Faith in God is the starting point and the foundation of the rest of the verse.

# CHAPTER 7: SPEAK TO THE MOUNTAIN

Let's review what Jesus said.

> [22] *"Have faith in God," Jesus answered.*
> [23] *"Truly I tell you, if anyone says to this mountain, 'Go, throw yourself into the sea,' and does not doubt in their heart but believes that what they say will happen, it will be done for them* (Mark 11:22-23).

This is a powerful and controversial passage of Scripture. We must remember that Jesus said, "Have faith in God." That is our starting point, our relationship with God. Then he tells the disciples of a potential power that is available to them, speaking to the mountain. What is a mountain? Was Jesus talking about a literal mountain? I don't think so. He was talking about obstacles in our lives that are beyond our ability to overcome. Because of our relationship with God, we see the obstacles that He sees, not just the ones that we see.

Why is speaking to the mountain important?

- It helps us identify obstacles or mountains in our lives. Mountains are those things that stand against what God wants to do.
- It helps us focus on the issues that are there rather than ignoring them.
- It helps us depend on God to help us overcome.
- Confession refocuses your life on God's truth, not your feelings or emotions.
- Speaking energizes us towards a goal. We see it all the time in sports and business. If you don't have a goal, then you don't know where you are headed.

117

- Speaking is standing up against what is going wrong in your life.

There is a spiritual component to speaking. Jesus says, "[7] If you remain in me and my <u>words</u> remain in you, ask whatever you wish, and it will be done for you. [8] This is to my Father's glory, that you bear much fruit, showing yourselves to be my disciples" (John 15:7-8).

In the first part of this passage, Jesus reminds us of the ongoing relationship, remaining in Him, that is required to expect answered prayer. Numerous Scriptures equate a vibrant relationship with Jesus as mandatory to receiving from God. Then and only then can you "ask whatever you wish, and it will be done for you."

Think of it this way. I have grandkids. I love my grandkids. They bring me so much joy. Each day is a new adventure with them. I want to do stuff for them. I want to spend time with them and buy them stuff. When I go to the store, my wife and I are thinking about the grandkids. "This would be so cute on him" or "She would love this." One of the things that keeps me from buying things for them is when they have a bad attitude or are unappreciative about what I have done for them. From whom do you think I got those feelings? That's right, God. He doesn't like it when we are ungrateful for what He has done for us. He doesn't like it when we have bad attitudes and complain; it hinders our prayers.

Jesus said it was to His Father's glory that we bear much fruit. What is fruit? Certainly, answered prayer is. Fruit is an indication of our discipleship.

The Apostle Paul gives us more information about prayer when he writes,

> *⁶ Do not be anxious about anything, but in every situation, by prayer and petition, <u>with thanksgiving</u>, present your requests to God. ⁷ And the peace of God, which transcends all understanding, will guard your hearts and your minds in Christ Jesus* (Phil. 4:6-7).

Paul tells us to thank God for the answer <u>before</u> we see the answer. By thanking God, we are acknowledging that God can answer our prayers. It is a faith statement.

Certainly, a person can pray quietly so that only God can hear them, but speaking out loud is more powerful because words are powerful and do something inside and outside of us. When we speak negative words, they reinforce the negative. Words like, "I can't do this," or "I'll never be able to ..." reinforces the negative we spoke inside of us causing the negative to be a stronger force for us to overcome. In the same way, positive words chip away at the negative attitude that tries to control us. Additionally, words are fruit that show what is growing inside of us. Jesus speaking to a group of people, including Pharisees says,

> *³³ "Make a tree good and its fruit will be good, or make a tree bad and its fruit will be bad, for a tree is recognized by its fruit. ³⁴ You brood of vipers, how can you who are evil say anything good? For the mouth speaks what the heart is full of. ³⁵ A good man brings good things out of the good stored up in him, and an evil man brings evil things out of the evil stored up in him. ³⁶ But I tell you that everyone will have to give account on the day of judgment for every <u>empty word</u> they have spoken. ³⁷ For by*

*your <u>words</u> you will be acquitted, and by your words you will be condemned"* (Matt. 12:33-37).

Jesus gives us so much to consider. We must give an account of our empty words. Empty words don't accomplish anything. Words acquit or condemn us because words are powerful and can change the direction of our lives. I am writing this as a student of the Word of God considering how my words affect me. It is so easy for me to become negative and see problems rather than what God's Word says about me. That is why Paul tells us to renew our minds in Romans 12. When we get our thinking right, our speech will change. When our speech changes, we will see how God works in our lives.

In his Sermon on the Mount, Jesus encourages us to refuse to worry about life, but to put Him first (Matt. 6:31-34).

In this example, Jesus points out that a person can verbalize what he or she is thinking by saying "What shall we eat?" This goes back to the previous Scripture where Jesus tells us that the mouth speaks what the heart is full of. The person is saying that they are worried about things. Jesus is telling us to not worry but seek God first. Jesus' emphasis is prioritizing seeking and building one's relationship God. That is central to understanding how God works in our lives and why He allows mountains. Here are a few things to consider.

## Why Mountains?

Why does God allow mountains in our lives? Because He wants us to learn to climb mountains— or to remove them or blow them up—with faith in God. God wants us to grow in our ability to endure and overcome struggles with the attitude of perseverance.

Why does Jesus tell us to speak to the mountain? Speaking is an important aspect of faith. The secular world understands the importance of saying out loud your goals. For example, "I am going to be the best salesperson in my division." Of course, a person's action must match their confession, but confession puts us on the trail to where we want to go. It makes us face the opposition of our present reality. It makes us face the opposition of people that stand against us, whether intentionally or inadvertently. It also helps us to direct our energy and align it with what is needed to overcome the mountain.

Speaking to the mountain also has to do with authority that God wants you to use. In the garden of Eden, Adam had authority over the garden. When he disobeyed God's only command, he gave his authority to the devil. Jesus took it back on the cross. Let's review some biblical examples.

In Matthew 4, we see Jesus speaking to the mountain. The mountains were temptations. The three temptations were very real to Jesus, but Jesus fought them with Scripture showing us how we should battle temptations. To use Scripture, we need to know it and that requires study. As stated earlier, Paul writes to Timothy encouraging him to be a good worker and study and correctly interpret Scripture (2 Tim. 2:15). We must study to understand what the Word says. We must study to show God we are serious about being a disciple. There is no shortcut.

When fighting the mountain of temptation, James weighs in writing, "Submit yourselves, then, to God. Resist the devil, and he will flee from you. ⁸ Come near to God and he will come near to you" (James 4:7-8a). We are no match for the devil on our own. However, when we submit to God, we are empowered to overcome. But temptation must be resisted. Mentally resisting is good, but verbally resisting is more powerful because we are resisting when we speak up. We are making our mind agree with the idea that we are resisting the temptation. But we are not tackling our struggles alone. We are using authority that God has given us.

## Authority

The author of Hebrews tells us,

> ¹⁴ *Therefore, since we have a great high priest who has* <u>*ascended*</u> *into heaven, Jesus the Son of God, let us hold firmly to the faith we profess.* ¹⁵ *For we do not have a high priest who is unable to empathize with our weaknesses, but we have one who has been* <u>*tempted*</u> *in every way, just as we are—yet he did not sin.* ¹⁶ *Let us then approach God's throne of grace with confidence, so that we may receive mercy and find grace to help us in our time of need* (Heb. 4:14-16).

In our battle to fight mountains, we need to realize the authority we have is because of what Jesus did. He is our high priest. He understands temptation, He understands trials, He understands sin, yet He didn't sin. Because of Him, we can boldly go before the Father and get help to overcome those mountains in our lives.

## Jesus Ascended

When talking about Jesus' ascension, the word translated "ascended" is in the perfect tense in the Greek language. In English we don't have anything like the perfect tense. In Greek, the perfect tense means that something happened in the past and caused continuing results into the future. In this case, ascended gives us the powerful implications of what ascension means.

- It means that Jesus isn't in the grave.
- It means that Jesus arose from the dead.
- It means that Jesus defeated the devil when He went to hades.[47]
- It means that Jesus preached to the dead while He was there.
- It means that Jesus led captivity captive and gave gifts to men (Eph. 4:8).
- It means that Jesus is restored to His proper place in heaven at the right hand of the Father.
- It means that Jesus is no longer the disrespected itinerant preacher but is the conquering king of the universe.
- It means that if you have accepted Jesus as your Lord and Savior, you have access to the Father through Jesus who is your High Priest.

Jesus intercedes to the Father for us. Jesus fights our battles. Jesus understands our weaknesses. This is a game changer. We have authority because of what Jesus did. We can approach Almighty God with our needs, and He has the resources to help us.

---

[47] Barclay, 273. Barclay differentiates between Jewish thought of hades and hell. He writes, "The difference is that hell is the place of the punishment of the wicked; Hades was the place where all the dead went."

I want to bring in another Scripture at this point to emphasize the huge impact that Jesus' death, resurrection, and ascension made. This is one of the most difficult passages in the New Testament to understand because of its reference to imprisoned spirits, Noah, and preaching to the dead. Scholars don't agree on its meaning, and there are at least four different views. Let's look at the first part and then the second part.

The Apostle Peter writes,

*[18] For Christ also suffered once for sins, the righteous for the unrighteous, to bring you to God. He was put to death in the body but made alive in the Spirit. [19] After being made alive, he went and made proclamation to the <u>imprisoned spirits</u>—[20] <u>to those who were disobedient</u> long ago when God waited patiently in the <u>days of Noah</u> while the ark was being built. In it only a few people, eight in all, were saved through water, [21] and this water symbolizes baptism that now saves you also—not the removal of dirt from the body but the pledge of a clear conscience toward God. It saves you by the resurrection of Jesus Christ, [22] who has gone into heaven and is at God's right hand—with angels, authorities and powers in submission to him (1 Pet. 3:18-22.)*

The point of this passage is that Jesus suffered, and suffering isn't always bad. Thomas Schreiner, a professor at Southern Baptist Theological Seminary in Louisville, writes,

*Now in vv. 18–22 Peter argued that Christ also traveled the pathway from suffering to glory. <u>Suffering, then, is not a sign of divine displeasure.</u> Precisely the opposite. Those who suffer for the Christ will be glorified as he was. The paragraph is a difficult one, but it has three main points. First, Christ suffered for the unrighteous to bring believers to God (v. 18). Second, by the power of the Spirit he was raised from the dead and proclaimed victory over demonic spirits* *(vv. 18–19). Finally, he is now exalted on high as the resurrected and ascended Lord and has subjected all demonic powers to himself (v. 22). The main point, then, is that believers have no need to fear that suffering is the last word, for they share the same destiny as their Lord, whose suffering has secured victory over all hostile powers. Believers, then, are akin to Noah. They are a small embattled minority in a hostile world, but they can be sure that, like Noah, their future is secure when the judgment comes. The basis of their assurance is their baptism, for in baptism they have appealed to God to give them a good conscience on the basis of the crucified (v. 18) and risen (v. 21) work of the Lord Jesus Christ.*[48]

The Apostle Peter has spoken much about suffering in his epistle. Suffering has a purpose. In Jesus' case, he suffered and died so that we could be free from sin. Peter also points out that Jesus proclaimed to imprisoned spirits. This is one of the areas of disagreements among scholars. Who or what are these spirits? Schreiner believes it is evil spirits. Basically, Jesus was doing a victory lap in front of the devil and his cronies.

Some believe that Jesus is preaching to lost people that haven't heard the gospel. That, coupled with verse 6 in the next chapter, gives some the idea that people are given a second chance to come to Jesus. I find this inaccurate for a couple of reasons. First, Jesus comments in a parable about the rich man and Lazarus show that there is a different place for the godless rich man and Lazarus. The rich man ends up being tormented in Hades while Lazarus is with Abraham. The rich man asks for relief from the

---

[48] Thomas R. Schreiner, *1 and 2 Peter, Jude*, vol. 37, The New American Commentary (Nashville: Broadman & Holman Publishers, 2003), 179–180.

torment but is told no by Abraham and reminded of how good he had it in his life. Furthermore, Abraham informs the rich man that "between us and you a great chasm has been set in place, so that those who want to go from here to you cannot, nor can anyone cross over from there to us" (Luke 16:26).

Then the rich man asks Abraham to send Lazarus to his brothers to warn them but once again Abraham refuses. He reminds the rich man that they have Moses and the prophets. The rich man responds,

> [30] "No, father Abraham," he said, "but if someone
> from the dead goes to them, they will repent."
> [31] He said to him, "If they do not listen to Moses and
> the Prophets, they will not be convinced even if someone
> rises from the dead" (Luke 16:30-31).

The decisions we make in this life are eternal. Jesus makes it clear that there are no second chances once you die. Also, if we could all change our minds, then eat, drink, and be merry because what we do in this life doesn't matter. The truth is that we will all stand before Almighty God and His son Jesus. No one will deny who Jesus is, but every knee will bow. That doesn't mean that anyone will have another opportunity to make amends for the life they lived. It is too late.

Let's look at the second half of the passage in 1 Peter.

> Therefore, since Christ suffered in his body, arm
> yourselves also with the same attitude, because whoever
> suffers in the body is done with sin. [2] As a result, they do not
> live the rest of their earthly lives for evil human desires, but
> rather for the will of God. [3] For you have spent enough time in
> the past doing what pagans choose to do—living in
> debauchery, lust, drunkenness, orgies, carousing and

126

*detestable idolatry. [4] They are surprised that you do not join them in their reckless, wild living, and they heap abuse on you. [5] But they will have to give account to him who is ready to judge the living and the dead. [6] For this is the reason the gospel was preached even to those who are now dead, so that they might be judged according to human standards in regard to the body, but live according to God in regard to the spirit* (1 Pet. 4:1-6).

Once again, suffering is a key component of this passage. Peter makes the statement that the person that suffers in the body is done with sin. Many that come to Christ throughout history suffer persecution. When that happens, a deep decision is made to live for God. Physical pain can be involved, as well as loss of family, life, and possessions, when a person decides to live for God. Unlike the "cheap grace[49]" that is often preached and seen in America, a price is paid to live for God. When that happens, sin loses its appeal. Eternity becomes the focus rather than this life because this life and eternity have already been compared and eternity is found to be more valuable.

The point of this passage in 1 Peter is that Jesus died, arose, and ascended to heaven. The devil was defeated, and victory was won for believers.

---

[49] Dietrich Bonhoeffer, *The Cost of Discipleship*, trans. Chr. Kaiser Verlage Munchen, R. H. Fuller, and Irmgard Booth (New York: Touchstone, 1995), 18,43. Bonhoeffer, coined the phrase "Cheap Grace." He said, "Cheap grace is the deadly enemy of our church. We are fighting today for costly grace." Bonhoeffer would be executed by the Nazis during WWII.

Let's return to our passage in Hebrews. Jesus our high priest has ascended and the passage also reminds us that he was tempted (Heb. 4:14-16).

## Jesus was tempted

The passage says that Jesus was tempted in every way just like us. It is so easy for us to think that we are the only ones who are going through the difficulty we are facing. We have the attitude like the saying I learned as a kid, "Nobody likes me, everybody hates me. I'm going to eat worms. Big fat juicy one, little, tiny, squirmy ones, I'm going to eat some worms." It sounds funny, but it is true. We think that everyone is against us and, worst of all, God is against us. But often we have tied his hands by the way we think and act. We need to grow up and put the blame where it belongs: on us and the devil. The devil tempts us and how we respond is significant.

It says that Jesus was tempted. Once again, the verb tempted is in the perfect tense. Jesus was tempted in the past with result continuing into the future. What are the results?

- It means Jesus understands.
- It means that Jesus has ever experienced what you are going through.
- It means you shouldn't feel sorry for yourself because there is a solution for your problem.
- It means that Jesus overcame temptation with Scripture and so can we.
- It means that when we pray to God, Jesus is interceding for us.

## Remain in Jesus

Jesus says more about a relationship with Him. "If you remain in me and my words remain in you, ask whatever you wish, and it will be done for you. [8] This is to my Father's glory, that you bear much fruit, showing yourselves to be my disciples" (John 15:7-8). This statement is revolutionary and powerful. Jesus speaks of results that we should see, fruit. It proves that we are Jesus' disciple.

But how do you remain in Jesus? Prayer and worship of God are part of it. But there is more. Foster whets our appetite writing, "The classical Disciplines of the spiritual life call us to move beyond surface living into the depths. They invite us to explore the inner caverns of the spiritual realm."[50] The apostle Paul was describing his adventure into knowing God in Philippians 3.

Part of the problem is that many don't believe that they can get that close to God. Only monks or a special few can really know God. Foster writes,

*God intends the Disciplines of the spiritual life to be for ordinary human beings; people who have jobs, who care for children, who wash dishes and mow lawns. In fact, the Disciplines are best exercised in the midst of our relationship with our husband or wife, our brothers and sisters, our friends and neighbors.*[51]

---

[50] Foster, 1.
[51] Ibid.

The Disciplines do not mean that we are relying solely on our own will to grow in the Lord. It is much like a farmer that prepares the soil and plants the seed but then is dependent on God to send the rain. Foster writes,

*"This is the way it is with the Spiritual Disciplines---they are a way of sowing to the Spirit. The Disciplines are God's way of getting us into the ground; they put us where he can work within us and transform us. By themselves the Spiritual Disciplines can do nothing; they can only get us to the place where something can be done."*[52]

Jesus verbally cursed the fig tree and it died. Then Jesus explained to the disciples what the cursing of the fig tree meant. Once again, it starts with having faith in God. He has just shown us how it works. He spoke to a fig tree, and it died. He is confirming the power of the spoken word by anyone, because now He tells us to speak to the mountain. He is exaggerating to get His point across. We would probably never have to ask a physical mountain to move. However, we will have to speak to many mountains or difficulties to be removed. He is telling us to have faith in God and speak to the different types of mountains. But our relationship with the Father will influence how strong we believe what we say and whether we doubt.

---

[52] Ibid., 7.

# CHAPTER 8: DOES NOT DOUBT

The problem with speaking to the mountain is that often there is a delay between the speaking and the results. What we do during the delay is important. That is where faith is required. We need to continue to feed on the Word of God to stay strong and not doubt.

There will be plenty of opportunities to doubt God's Word. Here are some of the reasons for doubt.

1. Don't Believe in God. Don't know who He is.

2. Don't Believe God is big enough to solve our problem.

3. Don't believe that God wants to solve the problem either because of His will or His timing. For the believer to not doubt, he or she needs to understand God's Will. For example, Abraham knew God told him he would have a son. Even then, he struggled to believe. Genesis shows us his struggle.

4. Don't believe that you are worthy of His response.

5. Don't believe that you are doing the necessary things to accomplish the result. For example, if we want to reach out to our community, we need to be out in the community. We must be obedient. Sometimes we don't put in the required prayer needed to find God's direction.

Faith requires action. For example, if you want a room painted, praying about it will not solve the problem. The paint and brush must be bought, and someone has to put the paint on the wall. Faith always requires doing something, even if that something is waiting in the Lord. Usually there is a step forward in faith that is required.

6. Don't believe God's Word. Somehow the enemy makes you doubt God at His Word. We must realize that it is the enemy that hinders the work of the Lord and not the Lord's delaying for some reason. My faith needs to be in the Lord and stand against the devil. <u>Doubt is irrational and doesn't look at the evidence. It is based in fear</u>. It looks at what can go wrong and not what can go right.

How long does it take to repair the damage when you have a faithless meltdown because of events not going as planned? I don't know, but one must re-engage one's faith in God as soon as possible. One must repent of doubting and recognize that the enemy hinders God's work. God is faithful and will forgive all unrighteousness (I John 1:9).

I refer you back to chapter 5 to review the difference between doubt and unbelief. Also in that section, I discuss James' understanding of faith versus doubt and the role that perseverance plays in it. Keep in mind from that discussion that doubts greatly hinders your prayers and your walk with the Lord. James further enforces the power of faith in action when he writes,

> [15] *And the prayer offered in faith will make the sick person well; the Lord will raise them up. If they have sinned, they will be forgiven.* [16] *Therefore confess your sins to each other and pray for each other so that you may be healed. The prayer of a righteous person is powerful and effective* (James 5:15-16).

Faith makes prayer work. So how do we grow in our faith? Some of this was discussed when looking at Abraham's life. "Does not doubt" is very similar to "Being fully persuaded" as discussed in Chapter 5. But I want to bring in some of Jesus' teaching on faith. Faith was the topic of discussion between the disciples and Jesus. Like us, they struggled with understanding how faith works and how you can get enough faith.

> *⁵ The apostles said to the Lord, "Increase our faith!"*
>
> *⁶ He replied, "If you have faith as small as a mustard seed, you can say to this mulberry tree, 'Be uprooted and planted in the sea,' and it will obey you. ⁷ "Suppose one of you has a servant plowing or looking after the sheep. Will he say to the servant when he comes in from the field, 'Come along now and sit down to eat'? ⁸ Won't he rather say, 'Prepare my supper, get yourself ready and wait on me while I eat and drink; after that you may eat and drink'? ⁹ Will he thank the servant because he did what he was told to do? ¹⁰ So you also, when you have done everything you were told to do, should say, 'We are unworthy servants; we have only done our duty.' "* (Luke 17:5-10).

At first glance, this passage seems a little bit odd. The disciples ask Jesus to teach them about faith. He tells them that they don't need much and then tells them about a servant. What was He trying to teach us? It is not the amount of faith that we need but the kind of faith...like a mustard seed. Leon Morris, an Australian scholar who edited and wrote for Tyndale New Testament Commentaries, wrote, "It is not so much great faith that is required as faith in a great God."[53] Morris is emphasizing, like Jesus, that it is not the size of our faith but in whom are faith is.

Norval Geldenhuys, a minister and scholar of the Dutch Reformed Church of South Africa, believes the preceding conversation about forgiveness revealed to the disciples their need for more faith. He writes,

> "The foregoing pronouncements impressed the
> disciples profoundly with the severe demands made
> upon them, and they feel spontaneously that they will
> require supernatural grace and divine strength in order
> so to live that they may avoid offending others and
> always be prepared to forgive the repentant. So they ask
> the Savior to give them greater faith–the faith that will
> make them spiritually stronger, and enable them to act
> as He has just commanded them to do.[54]

Geldenhuys also emphasizes the need for a "Vigorous, living faith." He continues, "If the disciples had had faith of the same quality of life and vigour, no problem or task would have been too difficult for them."[55] In his comments about the servant that follows, he writes,

> When believers have received the gift of a living
> faith and as a result are able to perform glorious things
> in His service, there is a great danger that they may
> become self-satisfied and may think themselves entitled
> to special marks of honour. Such an attitude, however, is
> quite wrong and sinful.[56]

---

[53] Leon Morris, *Luke: An Introduction and Commentary, Tyndale New Testament Commentaries,* vol. 3, (Downers Grove, IL: InterVarsity Press, 1988), 273.

[54] Norval Geldenhuys, *The Gospel of Luke, The International Commentary on the New Testament* (Grand Rapids, MI: W.M. B. Eerdmans Publishing Co. Reprinted, 1988), 432.

[55] Ibid.

[56] Ibid., 432-433.

Morris also warns of spiritual pride. He writes,

> *When people have such faith they may be
> tempted to spiritual pride. Jesus teaches humility by
> referring to standard practice with slaves. At the end of
> the day's work the master does not call the slave to have
> dinner... Rather he calls on the slave to serve him while
> he eats. And he does not thank the slave for doing what
> he is told. That is no more than his duty. So with God's
> servants ('slaves').*[57]

We are God's slaves. To sum up, it is not so much the size of the faith, but the faith in the big God. Also, don't get puffed up when God does use you, but remember we are slaves of Christ.

I also notice another aspect of this passage. It isn't so much the size of the faith but using that vibrant faith to be obedient to do what God wants us to do. If you do God's will, then you will have enough of whatever you need to complete the task.

You don't see the New Testament church going around and confessing this or that. You see them doing battle with the enemy of our souls often at great price to themselves. Paul ascended to the third heaven in one of his visions and had signs and wonders follow him, but he was still beaten many times and shipwrecked multiple times. The Prosperity Gospel focuses on what you can get and not what you can give. It focuses on authority and not obedience. Because of that, it is out of balance centering on the rewards of this life rather than building one's treasure in heaven.

---

[57] Morris, 274.

# CHAPTER 9: BELIEVES WHAT WE SAY

Much has been written about believing what you say will happen. Charles Capps wrote an entire book called *The Tongue a Creative Force*[58]. In his book, Capps highlights many Scriptures that emphasis the importance of what we say. He even tells his own personal story about how God fixed his farming business through his spoken word combined with faith.[59] He goes so far as to say, "Prayer is your <u>legal right</u> to use faith filled words to bring God on the scene in your behalf, or for another that your joy may be full."[60] Then he quotes Jesus speaking, "If you remain in me and my words remain in you, ask whatever you wish, and it will be done for you. 8 This is to my Father's glory, that you bear much fruit, showing yourselves to be my disciples" (John 15:7-8). It makes the Father happy when we bear much fruit.

Foster takes a little different approach to prayer than Capps. He doesn't say anything about prayer being our legal right, but he does believe that our prayers should be answered. When they are not answered, there is a reason. He believes that we learn to pray through trial and error. In his study of prayer, he cut out all the Jesus' teaching dealing with prayer and studied them. He writes,

> *When I could read Jesus' teaching on prayer at one sitting, I was shocked. Either the excuses and*

---

[58] Charles Capps, *The Tongue a Creative Force* (Tulsa, OK: Harrison House, 1976).

[59] Ibid., 51.

[60] Ibid., 10.

*rationalizations for unanswered prayer I had been taught were wrong, or Jesus' words were wrong. I determined to learn to pray so that my experience conformed to the words of Jesus rather than try to make his words conform to my impoverished experience.[61]*

Surprisingly, Foster observed that neither Jesus, nor the apostles, nor prophets concluded prayers with "If it be thy will." Foster believes they knew God's will before they prayed. He believes prayers should be decisive, though he admits there are times when we ask for God's guidance or will in our lives.[62]

In Foster's quest to learn to pray, he likened prayer to a TV set. If a TV isn't working, then one doesn't consider the transmission from the station as not existing but tries to figure out what is wrong with the set. It could be something like the plug-in. He used this illustration over 25 years ago, so it is somewhat dated even though cable does go out from time to time, but the point is well taken. Whatever the problem is, it takes effort to diagnose what the problem is. The same is true of prayer. If your prayers aren't being answered, then something is hindering it. It doesn't mean that God doesn't answer prayer.[63]

Your prayers not being answered could have to do with your motives. James writes, "When you ask, you do not receive, because you ask with wrong motives, that you may spend what you get on your pleasures"

---

[61] Foster, 36.
[62] Ibid., 37.
[63] Ibid., 38-39.

(James 4:3). James has a great deal to say about worldly motives and friendship with the world. It is imperative that we examine our motives to better understand what is driving us and allow the Holy Spirit to illuminate our hearts and show us where we should change.

Believing what we say is greatly influenced by the condition of our hearts. If we are negative in our hearts, it will come out. Let me remind you again of what Jesus said.

> For the mouth speaks what the heart is full of.
> [35] A good man brings good things out of the good stored up in him, and an evil man brings evil things out of the evil stored up in him. [36] But I tell you that everyone will have to give account on the day of judgment for every empty word they have spoken. [37] For by your words you will be acquitted, and by your words you will be condemned" (Matt. 12:34b-37).

I need to briefly mention what should take place in a person's life when he or she messes up. I must admit, I speak from experience. I know how it is to try so hard to grow in my relationship with the Lord and then get blind-sided and respond inappropriately. What do we do when that happens? Whenever we sin, we shouldn't stay in that state of mind. Have we lost our salvation? No, but we have placed a barrier between us and God, and it needs to be fixed. How do we fix it? John tells us how. He tells us to go to God and confess our sins. When we do that God forgives our sins and mends that relationship between us and God (1 John 1:9).

We need to confess to God what we have done. The devil wants us to brood around in self-pity and justification, making excuses for our actions. That does not solve anything. We need to admit our sins and God will forgive us and cleanse us. It is simple but hard to do as our pride does not want us to admit we were wrong. In our effort to live all out for God, we will make mistakes, and when we do, we need to get things right with God as soon as possible.

What does this have to do with believing what we say? A great deal, because we always need to allow the Holy Spirit the room to illuminate where we are falling short, whether it is our speech or actions. Both our speech and our actions are driven, as Jesus said, from what is inside of us. Foster deals with change on the inside and out in his chapter on simplicity. He writes, "The Christian Discipline of simplicity is an inward reality that results in an outward life-style."[64] The way Foster tackles simplicity will almost certainly make you uncomfortable. It did me. He attacks the consumer-driven American culture writing, "Contemporary culture lacks both the inward reality and the outward life-style of simplicity. We must live in the modern world, and we are affected by its fractured and fragmented state."[65] He further explains,

> *Because we lack a divine Center our need for security has led us into an insane attachment to things. We really must understand that the lust for affluence in contemporary society is psychotic. It is psychotic because it has completely lost touch with reality. We crave things we neither need nor enjoy.*[66]

---

[64] Ibid., 79.
[65] Ibid., 80.
[66] Ibid.

According to Foster, our consumer driven society has shamed us into buying stuff we don't need. "Covetousness we call ambition. Hoarding we call prudence. Greed we call industry."[67]

For our words to have the proper effect, we need to be counter-cultural. That will only happen if we understand the spiritual world in which we live. The apostle Paul gives us much of what we understand about spiritual warfare. He tells us that our weapons are not what we normally think of, such as guns and knives, but are divine and tear apart strongholds (2 Cor. 10:3-5). In that passage, notice that he mentions demolishing arguments and taking captive our thoughts. Our words and thoughts do matter. We need to pay attention to what we think and speak.

In Paul's description of the armor of God, he lists the sword of the Spirit, which is the Word of God (Eph. 6:17). Speaking God's Word has power. Jesus demonstrated that when He fought temptation in the wilderness by quoting the Old Testament. (Matt. 4:1-11).

Words can also affect the outcome of our prayers. What our heart is full of can fight against our prayer. Capps gives us three statements:

- The spirit world is controlled by the Word of God.
- The natural world is to be controlled by man speaking God's Words.
- The spoken Word of God is creative power.[68]

Whether you agree with Capps or not, Jesus' statement sure gives credibility to the idea that we should examine our speech. Jesus warns that by your

---

[67] Ibid., 81.
[68] Capps, 8.

words you will be acquitted or condemned. Does our speech agree with God's Word or not? Where can we improve?

Capps continues, "Therefore, even the words of our prayers should be chosen carefully and spoken accurately. We have often prayed, 'Lord I have prayed and it's not working out. The devil has defeated me.' "[69] According to Capps, this would hinder your prayer.

So much more could be said about believing what you say. I must confess that I am convicted as I write this because self-examination reveals weaknesses in my own speech. For example, how does our speech affect our country and politics? How does it affect the war in Ukraine or the Chinese plans for military action in Taiwan, or the security of our country with our open border? Our world is faced with serious challenges, and basically, I am asking if my Christian faith can make a difference in the challenges in our world. The answer is absolutely yes. But often my speech does not reflect that but focuses on the seriousness of the situation without regard to God's ability to change things.

How does this work with cancer or sickness? When I first started going to the hospital for chemo, I parked at the far end of the parking lot, regardless of the weather. When I got out of my truck, I would put a smile on my face and be pleasant to anyone with whom I came in contact. The quarter of a mile I walked gave me a chance to think about how thankful I was to be alive and focus on what was right with my life and not what was

---

[69] Ibid.

wrong. My mental attitude is absolutely essential to my survival. God is my source of my daily healing.

So, what is the answer or strategy for solving world problems? Before I answer that, I am reminded of something David Wilkerson said 50 years ago in his book *The Vision*.[70] He gave compelling prophecies about the state of the world and things that were going to happen. Some have already happened. As God revealed to Wilkerson in his vision, it disturbed him. But God comforted Wilkerson with five words and they still apply today; "God has everything under control."

Our starting point for figuring out where we fit into the puzzle of life is to remember that we are only a small part of the puzzle and "God has everything under control." With that in mind, we must understand that God's overall plan is in progress. We are not privy to understanding all about that process. Jesus gives us some clues in Matthew 24 about the end times when He talks about wars and rumors of war, false Messiahs, the prophecy of Daniel, signs and wonders, and the difficulty of the times. The times end with the second coming of Christ. Jesus warns his listeners, "Therefore keep watch, because you do not know on what day your Lord will come" (Matt. 24:42).

Jesus does tell us that we can look at the signs to know that the end is near.

*[32] "Now learn this lesson from the fig tree: As soon as its twigs get tender and its leaves come out, you*

---

[70] David Wilkerson, *The Vision: A Terrifying Prophecy of Doomsday That is Starting to Happen Now!* (Spire Book, 1973).

142

*know that summer is near. [33] Even so, when you see all these things, you know that it is near, right at the door. [34] Truly I tell you, this generation will certainly not pass away until all these things have happened. [35] Heaven and earth will pass away, but my words will never pass away* (Matt. 24:32-35).

Israel became a country again in 1948 and most scholars feel that historic event marked the end of the times of the Gentiles about which Jesus spoke. "Jerusalem will be trampled on by the Gentiles until the times of the Gentiles are fulfilled" (Luke 21:24b). The clock is ticking rapidly towards Jesus' return. It doesn't matter whether you and I agree or not, everything is going according to God's plan. If you do believe, however, then you will live your life differently. That will start with your understanding that "God has everything under control."

We are instructed to pray for our leaders. "I urge, then, first of all, that petitions, prayers, intercession and thanksgiving be made for all people—[2] for kings and all those in authority, that we may live peaceful and quiet lives in all godliness and holiness" (1 Tim. 2:1-2). We are to believe that our prayers and what we say make a difference in what our leaders do. Paul wrote this during the Roman Empire. Those were difficult times, but he must have felt that his prayers and what he said made a difference and so do ours. So, as we discuss our world events, discuss them in light of God's hand working towards His goals and continue to uplift world leaders, especially our country's leaders.

143

# CHAPTER 10: IT WILL BE DONE FOR YOU

"It will be done for you," is a powerful statement. If you have faith centered in God and speak to a mountain without doubting because somehow you believe what you say happens, it will be done for you. Who will do it? How will it be done? It doesn't say, but this is the power of God in operation. But it is not like we are little gods running around commanding God and His spiritual forces to do our bidding. It is more complicated than that. It requires a relationship with God.

God's Will is also involved. John writes, "This is the confidence we have in approaching God: that if we ask anything according to his will, he hears us. [15] And if we know that he hears us—whatever we ask—we know that we have what we asked of him" (1 John 5:14-15).

Here are a couple of things to consider. This passage says nothing about doubt, but it does tell us how to get confidence by asking according to God's will.

## Asking anything according to His will.

How do we find out about what His will is? By reading and studying His Word. Any directive we think God has given us in prayer should be vetted according to the Word of God. Here's a bad example: Someone will say something like, "God wants me to be happy." Then based on this, they leave their spouse and their children for another person. A careful study of God's Word would show a person that God doesn't like divorce and that marriage is more than a person simply feeling happy. It is about commitment to family and one's spouse. God wants you to be obedient and holy, which will bring happiness in God.

We know, for example, that God tells us to pray to the Lord of the harvest for helpers in the harvest (Matt. 9:38). Praying that prayer would be according to God's will and therefore we know that God hears us and will answer our prayer.

## God hears us

The challenge comes when we don't see an answer right away. Daniel, when praying about Jeremiah's prophecy regarding the people of Israel returning home, fasted and prayed. The angel Gabriel arrived with an answer saying, "As soon as you began to pray, a word went out, which I have come to tell you, for you are highly esteemed..." (Dan. 9:23a). Scripture doesn't tell us how long Daniel waited for the answer. However, in the next chapter, Daniel prays and fasts for three weeks before he receives an answer. An angel appeared.

> [11] *He said, "Daniel, you who are highly esteemed, consider carefully the words I am about to speak to you, and stand up, for I have now been sent to you." And when he said this to me, I stood up trembling.*

> [12] *Then he continued, "Do not be afraid, Daniel. Since the first day that you set your mind to gain understanding and to humble yourself before your God, your words were heard, and I have come in response to them.* [13] *But the prince of the Persian kingdom resisted me twenty-one days. Then Michael, one of the chief princes, came to help me, because I was detained there with the king of Persia* (Dan. 10:11-13).

This Scripture gives us a little insight into the spiritual battle that rages in the heavenly realms that we can't normally see. When we get to Heaven, we can ask the Father whether Daniel's 21-day fast affected the outcome of the prayer somehow. Did it speed up the answer or would it have come anyway? I am inclined to believe it did speed up the answer because of a couple of examples Jesus gives us.

In His Sermon on the Mount, Jesus said, "Ask and it will be given to you; seek and you will find; knock and the door will be opened to you. For everyone who asks receives; the one who seeks finds; and to the one who knocks, the door will be opened" (Matt. 7:7-8).

In verse seven, ask, seek, and knock are all imperatives or commands. Jesus expects us to have an active relationship with God that meets our needs. In verse eight, He gives us more details about our efforts to receive from God. When He says, asks, seeks, and knocks, He uses the present tense, which implies continuous action. In another words, we don't pray just once about something. We keep asking, seeking, and knocking. We are rewarded for our diligence in our actions. Jesus emphasizes this further in the next example.

> *Then Jesus told his disciples a parable to show them that they should always pray and not give up. ² He said: "In a certain town there was a judge who neither feared God nor cared what people thought. ³ And there was a widow in that town who kept coming to him with the plea, 'Grant me justice against my adversary.'*
>
> *⁴ "For some time he refused. But finally he said to himself, 'Even though I don't fear God or care what people think, ⁵ yet because this widow keeps bothering*

*me, I will see that she gets justice, so that she won't eventually come and attack me!' "*

*⁶ And the Lord said, "Listen to what the unjust judge says. ⁷ And will not God bring about justice for his chosen ones, who cry out to him day and night? Will he keep putting them off? ⁸ I tell you, he will see that they get justice, and quickly. However, when the Son of Man comes, will he find faith on the earth?"* (Luke 18:1-8).

Jesus told this parable so that His disciples would keep praying and not give up. That confirms to us that there are times when one prayer is not enough. It wasn't enough for the prophet Daniel, who prayed for 21 days, and it isn't enough for us either. Prayer is warfare. Our prayers are like bullets in a war with the enemy. It takes more than one bullet to win.

Some prayers, however, get immediate results. As you may recall from chapter 4, King Hezekiah brought about amazing reforms in Judah. In spite of all the good things he did, Sennacherib, the Assyrian king, came against him. When Sennacherib sent his threating letter, Hezekiah went into the temple and spread the letter out before God and prayed. God responded by sending a message to Isaiah and answered Hezekiah's prayer by striking Sennacherib's army and killing 185,000 soldiers. When Sennacherib returned home, his own sons killed him. What an answer to Hezekiah's prayer!

We don't know exactly how God answers our prayers, but He does. We need to pray according to God's Will and trust him to answer.

## Confidence we have received.

If we know that God hears us because we have asked according to His will, then we have confidence that we have received that for which we asked. Sometimes, however, we don't expect results. King Herod arrested James the brother of John and then had him put to death. Next, Herod arrested Peter and intended to kill him after the Passover, but the church prayed. In the middle of the night, the angel of the Lord led Peter out of jail. He went to the house where people were praying. The church was shocked to see Peter.

> *13 Peter knocked at the outer entrance, and a servant named Rhoda came to answer the door. 14 When she recognized Peter's voice, she was so overjoyed she ran back without opening it and exclaimed, "Peter is at the door!"*
>
> *15 "You're out of your mind," they told her. When she kept insisting that it was so, they said, "It must be his angel."*
>
> *16 But Peter kept on knocking, and when they opened the door and saw him, they were astonished. 17 Peter motioned with his hand for them to be quiet and described how the Lord had brought him out of prison. "Tell James and the other brothers and sisters about this," he said, and then he left for another place (Acts 12:13-17).*

God wants to answer our prayers in ways beyond our imagination. Let's examine a few more things about prayer in the next chapter.

# CHAPTER 11: WHATEVER YOU ASK FOR IN PRAYER

When we have a relationship with God that results in faith in God, it affects how we live. What we say is different because we have been changed on the inside. We are able to speak to our mountains and slay the giants. Somehow, God answers our prayers using resources that we don't see. But Jesus wasn't done yet in this passage. He has more to say about prayer, "Therefore I tell you, whatever you ask for in prayer, believe that you have received it, and it will be yours" (Mk. 11:24). Jesus has talked about speaking to the mountains and now He is telling us to believe when we pray. It doesn't do anyone any good when our prayers aren't answered. God wants to answer our prayers. As we talked about earlier, we need to pray with the right motives, but we should expect our prayers to be answered.

## Forgiveness

Jesus brings in another component of prayer: forgiveness. Churches are loaded with people that are angry with each other. Churches split over the dumbest reasons and the devil laughs at us. Christian marriages split because of unforgiveness. We are supposed to be the light of the world. Instead, we are an embarrassment to God because we don't forgive each other. Look what Jesus says. "And when you stand praying, if you hold anything against anyone, forgive them, so that your Father in heaven may forgive you your sins" (Mark 11:25). You want your sins forgiven, then forgive others.

149

There are many reasons that we don't want to forgive others. The main reason is that we feel others have wronged us. They somehow took away our rights. Maybe that is true, but that is still no excuse for not forgiving people. Jesus gives us several more examples. In the Lord's prayer Jesus warns us to forgive.

*[12] And <u>forgive us our debts,</u>*
*<u>as we also have forgiven our debtors</u>.*
*[13] And lead us not into temptation,*
*but deliver us from the evil one.'*
*[14] For if you forgive other people when they sin against you, your*
*heavenly Father will also forgive you. [15] But if you do not forgive others*
*their sins, your Father will not forgive you sin* (Matt. 6:12-15).

Jesus prays to the Father to forgive us as we forgive others. Then He mentions again that the Father will not forgive us if we don't forgive others. Forgiving others isn't an option but a command. There is a reason that God requires us to forgive. First, physically our bodies don't do too well when we harbor unforgiveness. Amanda Rowett, a licensed mental health counselor writes, "Just as a physical wound becomes infected if left unattended, so an emotional wound can become contaminated with feelings of resentment, bitterness, and revenge without the healing of forgiveness."[71] Rowett continues,

*Unforgiveness is a state of emotional and mental*
*distress that results from a delayed response in forgiving*
*an offender. It is characterized by indignation,*
*bitterness, and a demand for punishment or restitution.*

---

[71] Amanda Rowett, "The Prison of Unforgiveness: A Christian Counselor's Perspective on Forgiveness," Bellevue Christian Counseling, April 14, 2015; https://bellevuechristiancounseling.com/articles/the-prison-of-unforgiveness

*Unforgiveness creates a domino effect that negatively impacts every part of us, including our emotions, thoughts, behaviors, body, spirit, and relationships. With unforgiveness, time does not heal all wounds—in fact, time further worsens and infects emotional pain. Unforgiveness is like carrying around a huge weight. The longer we carry a grudge, the heavier the burden becomes. In the absence of a timely response, the roots of unforgiveness only go deeper, further entangling us. In sum, feeding on unforgiveness is toxic.[72]*

Nelson Mandela spent over 25 years in jail in South Africa for being an anti-apartheid activist.[73] Mandela certainly had a "right" from a human perspective to hold unforgiveness because of the way he was treated, but he recognized the destructive nature of unforgiveness. Rowett quotes him saying, "Hating someone is drinking poison and expecting the other person to die from it."[74]

Rowett has three articles on unforgiveness that are well worth reading. A final thought from her cites the medical problems that unforgiveness brings.

*Unforgiveness also compromises our physical health. Research has shown that unforgiveness is connected to high blood pressure, weakened immune systems, reduced sleep, chronic pain, and cardiovascular problems. Because unforgiveness hinders the body's ability to heal,*

---

[72] Ibid.

[73] Nelson Mandela Foundation, "Biography of Nelson Mandela," Accessed Dec. 19, 2022, https://www.nelsonmandela.org/content/page/biography.

[74] Rowett.

151

*forgiveness exercises are now being included in cancer treatment plans for patients.*[75]

Beyond the physical benefits of forgiving, there are other reasons. Forgiveness disarms people. Our sinful nature wants to punish people who treat us wrong. That is not God's way. When we show forgiveness to those that have wronged us, we open the door for God's love to change someone's life. A good example of this is found in Jesus' instruction to tell us to go the extra mile.

> [38] *You have heard that it was said, "Eye for eye, and tooth for tooth." [39] But I tell you, do not resist an evil person. If anyone slaps you on the right cheek, turn to them the other cheek also. [40] And if anyone wants to sue you and take your shirt, hand over your coat as well. [41] If anyone forces you to go one mile, go with them two miles. [42] Give to the one who asks you, and do not turn away from the one who wants to borrow from you* (Matt. 5:38-43).

Everything about this passage goes against what my sinful nature wants to do. I want an eye for an eye. I want to get even. I want revenge. "Do not resist an evil person." Are you kidding? If someone slaps me, I want to punch back. I am concerned about my rights.

Then Jesus brought out the "go the extra mile" line. This had to cause a huge number of emotions in the Jewish people because Jesus was referring to a law that required the Jewish people to carry stuff for a conquering Roman soldier for a mile. Picture working at your shop building furniture to sell, and a Roman soldier tells you to carry his stuff. You must stop

---

[75] Ibid.

working and carry this guy's stuff for a mile. It is a mile out and a mile back. Your work stops. It affects your delivery schedule and literally costs you money.

As you start walking with the soldier, neither one of you says anything. You are angry and the Roman soldier isn't happy about being in what he considers a primitive land. But then you remember what Jesus says about going the extra mile. When you get to the mile turnaround, you tell the soldier that you will go another mile. He is stunned. No one has ever done that for him. He doesn't know what to say. The soldier is disarmed. Any resistance he has towards you has been reduced.

As you begin the second mile, you begin talking. You find out that the soldier has a family and a new child he has never seen. He doesn't want to be there anymore than you want him to be there. What started out as a bitter relationship has worked into a friendship. It does amazing things to the soldier to find out that someone cares about him and his life. Over time, because you have gone the extra mile, you have a chance to tell him about your relationship with Jesus. This is an example of the power of forgiveness and how it can work. Allow the Holy Spirit to work in your life and show you how forgiveness can work in your life. Yes, it is time consuming to go the extra mile. Yes, it does mess up your schedule, but it works and brings about changes in people's lives.

# SECTION FOUR: HEALING

## CHAPTER 12: MATTHEW 8

Healing is an important subject for all of us. I have so many questions about healing. Does God want to heal me? Does God want me well? Are there hindrances to healing? Do I have enough faith? Am I good enough for God to heal me or are my sins keeping me from being healed? Is God trying to teach me something through my sickness? Jesus healed people, but does that mean He will heal me today in 2023? Is something holding me back?

For me, trusting God for healing is a challenge, but God has helped me to trust Him for the nine years I have dealt with cancer. I have much to learn, but Scripture has helped me to begin to understand God's view on sickness. Let's examine Matthew 8 & 9 which tell us much about healing.

### The Leper

Matthew Chapter Eight has some interesting insights into healing. Right away we see that Jesus is confronted by those that are sick.

*When Jesus came down from the mountainside, large crowds followed him. ² A man with leprosy came and knelt before him and said, "Lord, if you are willing, you can make me clean."*

*³ Jesus reached out his hand and touched the man. "I am willing," he said. "Be clean!" Immediately he was cleansed of his leprosy. ⁴ Then Jesus said to him, "See that you don't tell anyone. But go, show yourself to the priest and*

*offer the gift Moses commanded, as a testimony to them"*
(Matt. 8:1-4).

The man's question is what many of us want to ask Jesus, "Are you willing to heal me?" We know that God can heal us, but will He? We can come up with all kinds of reasons why we think God wouldn't want to heal us, such as our sinful life or our failure to do things that we know God wants us to do. Maybe we feel unworthy of His healing. None of this was brought into the equation by Jesus. He didn't ask the man about his spiritual life and if he had been living right. He didn't make him confess his sins and commit to living for God. He simply said, "I am willing."

Why is it so hard for us to receive from God? We are like Adam and Eve hiding in the garden of Eden from God. Our sins have shown us our nakedness and helplessness. It also shows us our need for forgiveness and a relationship with God. We need God to be Lord of our lives. Our lives are His. We should be living for Him.

Years ago, I was flying for a company. When I got to work that morning, there was a water leak in the hanger. There was a couple of inches of water on the floor. Right at that moment, I heard the Spirit of God ask me, "Does this bother you." "No," I thought, it didn't bother me. "Why?", He asked. Because I didn't own it, I realized. It wasn't my problem. I don't own my body either. I am God's property. He wants to keep my body working properly. He wants me well, so that I can better serve Him.

So, Jesus answered the leper, "I am willing, be clean." There are a number of key principles that we can draw from this passage. First, the man with leprosy went to Jesus. Second, Jesus responded with the answer, "I am willing." Jesus could have commented on the man's behavior or the difficulty of the disease to heal. The leper was asking Jesus for a miracle for Him to heal an incurable disease. Leprosy was a terrible disease that caused its victim to die a slow death separated from family and friends, but Jesus said, "I am willing, be clean."

Another question we must ask is, "Does God want us to be well?" Does this one episode represent His will for all of us. If he does want us to be well, then why are so many Christians sick? Is it because we don't have enough faith? I wish it were that simple.

There are hindrances to being healed. The way we treat our bodies, what we eat, lack of exercise, lack of rest, etc. I think that sometimes there are lessons to be learned in the middle of a sickness or a storm. I am reminded of a story about a blind man and what Jesus said to His disciples about the cause of a man's blindness.

*As he went along, he saw a man blind from birth.*
*[2] His disciples asked him, "Rabbi, who sinned, this man or his parents, that he was born blind?"*

*[3] "Neither this man nor his parents sinned," said Jesus, "but this happened so that the works of God might be displayed in him* (John 9:1-3).

This man had suffered all his life with no hope of ever seeing. Scripture doesn't tell us that he asked Jesus to heal him, but Jesus did. The man had to be obedient and go to the pool of Siloam. I have been to the pool of Siloam. It isn't much by our standards today. It is about the size of a small pool, but Jesus told him to wash there.

We don't know how far he had to go. It must have been difficult for him to find his way. What was he thinking during those minutes he was finding his way? "Am I going to be healed?" Maybe he was thinking about the things that he would be able to do. He would be able to work. Working would make him feel like he was a man and had value. He could have a family with children. He could run and play with them. The possibilities were endless. But he had to get to the pool. He also could have decided, "What's the use, Jesus isn't going to heal me?" Maybe he had never heard of Jesus. He could have not believed and disobeyed. The outcome would have been different.

This reminds me of another biblical story. The great Syrian commander Naaman had leprosy (2 Kings 5). He heard about the prophet in Israel that could heal him, so he set out to find him. When Naaman reached Elisha's house, Elisha didn't even come out to meet him. He sent a servant to tell him to wash seven times in the Jordan river. This upset Naaman so bad that he wasn't going to go to the Jordan, but his servants convinced him to be obedient. Once he washed seven times in the Jordan, he was healed.

Naaman had a couple of issues that could have kept him from being healed. The first one was pride. He thought that because of who he was, the prophet would do something special for him. He thought he deserved to be healed. He had to humble himself. Second, he had to be obedient. American Christians want to talk about rights that we have as a child of the King, but we don't want to talk about responsibilities and obedience.

Third, Naaman had to get beyond his preconceived ideas about the workings of God. He expected God to work through the prophet in a certain way. We have preconceived ideas of how God should do things, but God is creative and wants to work in new and fresh ways. Also, God has a different goal than we do. God's goal is for us to be like Jesus or made in His image. His goal is not for us to be comfortable.

Back to the story of the leper that Jesus heals. Notice that Jesus speaks to the disease, "Be clean!" Jesus doesn't pray, "Our Father in heaven, heal this man." He speaks to the leprosy. There is phenomenal power in Jesus' spoken word.

Look at what the book of Hebrews says about Jesus' Word. "The Son is the radiance of God's glory and the exact representation of his being, sustaining all things by his powerful word" (Heb. 1:3). It is important that we understand that Jesus is the exact representation of the Father. We want to know what God is like, so we should look at Jesus. We want to know what God thinks, so we should look at Jesus. Jesus sustains things by His powerful Word.

The question is, "How does Jesus' powerful word pertain to us and our confession?" Does what we say matter? Does it influence the outcome of our prayers? Does it influence the outcome of our sickness? I think it does...for several reasons. The first is because we are made with the image of God inside of us. We look like our daddy, God. There is an incredible human spirit that each of us has that wants to overcome and fight against the troubles we face. We hear about it all the time in the news. Someone overcame incredible odds physically to accomplish some great feat. It is the image of God inside of us that fights to bring about change in our situation.

Second, confession works. Years ago, I read a bunch of sales books which talked about the power of confessing your goals in sales or anything else. Speaking out loud our goals puts us on the road to accomplishing them. It helps us crystallize what we want, driving us to do tangible things to help us accomplish our goals. This is positive motivation, and it works.

Napoleon Hill wrote his great classic, *Think and Grow Rich*, in 1937. He was mentored and challenged by Andrew Carnegie to interview 500 millionaires and find the formula for success.[76] His formula, found in his book, starts with "The Power of Thought." In that chapter he tells the story of Edwin C. Barnes, who "thought" his way into a partnership with Thomas Edison.[77] If one continues reading the chapter titles, it is easy to see how the ideas conveyed could be life altering.

Confessing the Word of God is even more powerful. The mind has powerful ability to accomplish and overcome things. When you agree with the Word of God, you are agreeing with the Creator of the Universe, the one who set this whole thing up. We must interpret Scripture properly and be careful to read it in context. Too often, we read Scripture and, because we don't see the results that the Scripture seems to indicate, we give up and ignore the passage.

---

[76] Napoleon Hill, *Think and Grow Rich: The Landmark Bestseller—Now Revised and Updated for the 21st Century* (New York: Jeremy P. Tarcher/Penguin, 2005), xiv.

[77] Ibid., 1-4.

Hill has a chapter titled, "Persistence: The Sustained Effort Necessary to Induce Faith." He writes, "Willpower and desire, when properly combined, make an irresistible pair."[78] Hill recognizes the power of the will tied with desire to overcome helps a person achieve their goal. When we turn our wills towards Almighty God, determined to live for Him, there are even greater possibilities.

Rather than giving up when Scriptures don't seem to have the desired results, we should be determined to find out why we are not seeing the Scripture fulfilled in our lives. For example, Jesus says,

> *[12] Very truly I tell you, whoever believes in me will do the works I have been doing, and they will do even greater things than these, because I am going to the Father. [13] And I will do whatever you ask in my name, so that the Father may be glorified in the Son. [14] You may ask me for anything in my name, and I will do it* (John 14:12-14).

What a powerful statement. If we believe in Jesus, we can do greater works than Jesus did. Also, Jesus said we could "ask me for anything in my name, and I will do it." Wow! Why are we not seeing greater works? People explain by saying that now we have television and greater groups of people can know about Jesus, and that is true. We also have modern medicine and that helps fight disease and sickness. But I think that Jesus is talking about more. He tells us how in the first verse, "Whoever believes in me..."That

---

[78] Ibid., 175.

kind of relationship doesn't come with an occasional prayer. We must fight for it.

Jude urges us "To contend for the faith that was once for all entrusted to God's holy people" (Jude 3b). This was Jesus' physical brother writing this. He was there watching Jesus do miracles, along with the rest of his family, and he thought Jesus was crazy. Jesus' mother and brothers came to take him home because they didn't believe (Matt. 12: 46-50). It wasn't until after the resurrection they believed. To believe, then, we need to come to grips with the resurrected Jesus.

## Fasting

Serious growing in the Lord requires radical changes. Fasting is one way that we can bring about significant changes. When we fast, we are telling our bodies that they are not going to boss us around. We are taking charge of our lives and showing the Father that we mean business. Isaiah 58 gives us the best explanation of what we can expect from fasting. The first five verses tell us how not to fast. Then, starting with Verse 6, we are given some of the results to expect from a fast.

> *⁶ "Is not this the kind of fasting I have chosen:*
> *to loose the chains of injustice*
> *and untie the cords of the yoke,*
> *to set the oppressed free*
> *and break every yoke?*
> *⁷ Is it not to share your food with the hungry*
> *and to provide the poor wanderer with shelter—*
> *when you see the naked, to clothe them,*
> *and not to turn away from your own flesh and*
> *blood?*
> *⁸ Then your light will break forth like the dawn,*

161

*and your healing will quickly appear;*
*then your righteousness will go before you,*
*and the glory of the LORD will be your rear guard*
(Isa. 58:6-8).

I have listed five things for starters that fasting does.

## 1. Breaks Every Yoke

Verse six tells us that fasting breaks yokes. Yokes are those things that handcuff us and keep us from overcoming in our lives. It can be people in our lives that are addicted to things. It can be mountains that need to be climbed.

Fasting is a discipline that we should have in our lives. If you have medical issues and medicines to take, then fast only breakfast or lunch. The most important part is to make sure that you spend time praying and meditating on God's Word. Otherwise, you are just dieting.

## 2. Character Change

From Verse seven, we see people's character is changed through fasting. The person that is fasting is reaching out to others that have needs. Before fasting, they probably didn't care, but fasting changes your heart. Now you care about those in need. It helps you not turn away from your own flesh and blood. We all have family members that we don't want to talk to or have trouble with because for decades they have done nothing but cause problems. Fasting changes that.

I have seen identical twins that didn't talk to each other. The devil wants to tear marriages apart, tear families apart. Fasting and prayer can break the yoke and change you and me.

## 3. Healing

Verse eight says it will bring healing. Since I was diagnosed with multiple myeloma 9 years ago, I get a cancer magazine every quarter. Recently, it had an article in it that discussed fasting and cancer. According to the article, when a person fasts, normal human cells repair themselves. Cancer cells' sole purpose in life is to reproduce themselves. During a fast, they don't get the nutrients they need to keep reproducing themselves so they, in essence, reproduce themselves to their own destruction. Medical science is just figuring the benefits to fasting, but Isaiah wrote about this 2800 years ago. God's Word is true.

A recent study published in the National Library of Medicine showed the benefits of fasting for people with type 2 diabetes. It says, "The results from this pilot study indicate that short-term daily IF may be a safe, tolerable, dietary intervention in T2DM patients that may improve key outcomes including body weight, fasting glucose and postprandial variability.[79] "IF" means "Intermittent Fasting" and "T2DM" means Type 2 Diabetes Mellitus. Another article highlights 8 ways that fasting can help.

---

[79] Terra G. Arnason, Matthew W. Bowen, and Kerry D. Nansell, "Effects of intermittent fasting on health markers in those with type 2 diabetes: A pilot study World Journal of Diabetes" in National Library of Medicine: National Center for Biotechnical Information, 2017 April 15 8(4); 154-164, https://www.ncbi.nlm.nih.gov/pmc/articles/PMC5394735/

It says, "Fasting may provide several health benefits, including weight loss, improved blood sugar control, and decreased inflammation. It might also offer protection against certain conditions like cancer and neurodegenerative disorders."[80]

## 4. Direction

I have used fasting and prayer as a way to find God's plan for my life many times. The most amazing was when I was a young man seeking God's direction. There is so much to this story, but know this: God changed me and gave me clear direction. Fasting helps you to hear from God.

## 5. Provision

Verse eleven tells us that when you fast and pray God will satisfy your needs in a sun-scorched land. Most people aren't farmers today and don't think about draughts. It is so easy for us to turn on the water faucet. But during Old Testament times, if it didn't rain in Israel at the right times, not only did you not have water but you didn't have food because your crops failed. This passage promises that in the middle of sun-scorched land He will satisfy your needs. In another words, in a bad economy God will take care of you. That is the power of fasting.

---

[80] Amy Richter and Rachael Ajmera, "8 Health Benefits of Fasting, Backed by Science," Healthline, Updated on Mar 13, 2023, https://www.healthline.com/nutrition/fasting-benefits.

As a side note, before you fast, come up with a game plan. Know how long you plan to fast, decide on Scriptures you want to meditate on, and think about specific things that about which you are fasting and praying so that you can track the results of your fast.

Back to the story of the leper for a final thought. Jesus told the man to not tell anyone but go to show himself to the priest. The priest was the one that could declare the leper free of the disease through the best medical procedures of the day: observation. When God heals us, the medical profession should be able to confirm the healing.

In both parallel examples found in Mark and Luke, Jesus told the guy to not tell anyone but show himself to the priest. Both Mark and Luke record the man telling everyone that Jesus healed him so that Jesus could no longer enter the cities but had to go to lonely places to preach.

Mark records an interesting comment on Jesus' response to the Leper's original question, "If you are willing?" Mark says that Jesus was indignant. Rodney L. Cooper, an international speaker, former National Director of Promise Keepers, and professor at Gordon Conwell Theological Seminary in Charlotte, writes,

> *Instead of the leper keeping his distance from Jesus, as the law directed, he came directly to Jesus, fell on his knees, and cried out for Jesus to make him clean. This man was full of faith. He did not doubt Jesus' ability to heal him, but he was not sure of Jesus' desire to heal him. But he was willing to take the risk.*[81]

---

[81] Rodney L. Cooper, *Mark*, *Holman New Testament Commentary*, vol. 2 (Nashville, TN: Broadman & Holman Publishers, 2000), 15–16.

165

The NLT version says Jesus was filled with compassion. Cooper disagrees, writing,

> The phrase **filled with compassion** is probably better translated as "being angered." Jesus was probably angry because he recognized this foul disease as the work of Satan. Jesus' anger was not focused on the man and his desire for healing but on Satan, whose work he came to destroy.[82]

In conclusion, this story teaches us that Jesus is willing to heal us.

## The Centurion

The second example in Matthew 8 involves a Roman Centurion.

> [5]When Jesus had entered Capernaum, a centurion came to him, asking for help. [6] "Lord," he said, "my servant lies at home paralyzed, suffering terribly."
>
> [7] Jesus said to him, "Shall I come and heal him?"
>
> [8] The centurion replied, "Lord, I do not deserve to have you come under my roof. But just say the word, and my servant will be healed. [9] For I myself am a man under authority, with soldiers under me. I tell this one, 'Go,' and he goes; and that one, 'Come,' and he comes. I say to my servant, 'Do this,' and he does it."
>
> [10] When Jesus heard this, he was amazed and said to those following him, "Truly I tell you, I have not found anyone in Israel with such great faith. [11] I say to you that many will come from the east and the west, and will take their places at the feast with Abraham, Isaac and Jacob in the kingdom of heaven. [12] But the subjects of the kingdom

---

[82] Ibid., 16.

*will be thrown outside, into the darkness, where there will*
*be weeping and gnashing of teeth."*

*[13] Then Jesus said to the centurion, "Go! Let it be*
*done just as you believed it would." And his servant was*
*healed at that moment*(Matt. 8:5-13).

In this story, we see that Jesus is reaching out to a Roman soldier, a centurion. This man was part of the occupying miliary force in Israel. Often there were problems between the Jews and the Romans, but Jesus doesn't hesitate to go with the centurion. Jesus gives us a great example of how we should act towards those that treat us wrong: loving your neighbor.

The centurion, rather than having Jesus go with him, throws Him a curve ball when he tells Jesus that he is not worthy for Him to come into his home. He further surprises Jesus when he tells Jesus to just say the word and his servant would be healed. Then the centurion tells Jesus how he understands authority. Jesus comments that He had not found anyone in Israel with such great faith. Then Jesus tells the centurion, "Let it be done just as you believed it would."

Let's review what we learned:

- Healing is about authority. The centurion understood Jesus as someone that had the authority, the will, and the ability to heal his servant.
- Healing is about faith in God that He can heal us.
- Healing can be for someone else. The centurion believed for healing for his servant.

The centurion was one of two people that Jesus commended for their great faith. The other one was also a Gentile woman who interceded with

Jesus for her daughter. Because she wouldn't give up, Jesus told her she had great faith and her daughter was healed (Matt. 15:21-28). We need great faith to press into God when we face the most difficult situations and not give up. In the next section, we see God predicted the healings that Jesus would do.

### The Mother-in-law

This section starts out with Jesus' healing Peter's mother-in-law.

*[14] When Jesus came into Peter's house, he saw Peter's mother-in-law lying in bed with a fever. [15] He touched her hand and the fever left her, and she got up and began to wait on him.*

*[16] When evening came, many who were demon-possessed were brought to him, and he drove out the spirits with a word and healed all the sick. [17] This was to fulfill what was spoken through the prophet Isaiah:*

*"He took up our infirmities and bore our diseases"* (Matt. 8:14-17).

When Jesus healed Peter's mother-in-law, it shows Jesus' willingness to heal people regardless of their faith. He just healed her.

As the word gets out that Jesus is in town, sick people show up to be healed. Jesus drove out the spirits with a word and healed all the sick. Matthew presents this as a fulfillment of the prophecy found in Isaiah 53. This passage is one of the most powerful in the Bible because it shows over 700 years before it happened that God was planning Jesus' crucifixion.

Think about how incredible this prophecy is. Think about the changes that 700 years means. If we go back 700 years from now, we're in the dark ages. It was before America was discovered. There was no reformation, no printing press, and no modern conveniences like electricity, automobiles, airplanes, Internet, telephone, cell phones, TV, and railroads. That was before the European empires of Britain, Spain, and France existed and before an accurate way of ocean navigation had been invented. [83]

If you look back 700 years before the time of Christ, there were also huge changes. There was no Roman, Greek, or Medio-Persian empire. The Assyrian empire was thriving, and the Babylonian empire was about to start. Weapons such as the catapult wouldn't be developed until around 400BC.[84] Fighting was done with knives, spears, swords, bows and arrows for the most part.

The point is that God the Father was planning Jesus' life and death long before it happened. Therefore, He predicted the crucifixion, and He predicted the healing aspect of Jesus' ministry so that we could understand that Jesus is truly the Messiah. Does that mean that we can expect healing today? Or was that just when Jesus prayed on earth for people to be healed? James, the brother of Jesus, answered this question. He writes,

> [14] *Is anyone among you sick? Let them call the*
> *elders of the church to pray over them and anoint them*
> *with oil in the name of the Lord.* [15] *And the prayer*

---

[83] Dava Sobel, *Longitude: The True Story of a Lone Genius Who Solved the Greatest Scientific Problem of His Time* (London: Fourth Estate Limited, 1998),76. A fascinating book about solving the problem of where a ship was East and West or their longitude. John Harrison presented a mechanical solution with his H1 clock. He met resistance from the scientific community that felt the solution should be solved through an astronomical solution.

[84] Abby Colwell, Sun Eoh, Meghan Halpern, & Kate Shea, "Stone-Hurling Catapult, Greece 400BCE," Smith College Museum of Ancient Inventions, 1997-1998. https://www.smith.edu/hsc/museum/ancient_inventions/hsc11b.htm.

*offered in faith will make the sick person well; the Lord will raise them up* (James 5:14-15).

The prayer offered in faith will make the sick person well. Then James writes about the prophet Elijah and tells us that he was a human being just like us. It is so easy for us to think that we can never be used of God, but we have the Bible to give us examples of how God used ordinary men and women to do extraordinary things. Elijah was an example of that. Elijah wasn't an educated man as far as we know. He didn't have great possessions or resources. As we read about him, we find that he got depressed at times just like us. He had his own share of problems, but God used him because he was willing to be used and he was obedient.

James continues by telling us about Elijah's prayer to stop and start the rain (James 5:17-18). Elijah's prayers influenced the weather. Wow!!! He prayed those prayers to help deal with the sinful leadership of Ahab and Jezebel in obedience to God (1 Kings 17).

The point is that prayer for sickness still works. Capps writes,

*Faith will make prayer work. Prayer won't work without faith. Faith will work without prayer. Prayer is one of the means of releasing faith, so if we will line ourselves up with the Word of God, and release our faith when we pray, we will see the power of God come alive in our lives.*[85]

That sounds easy. Prayer plus faith equals healing. But what happens when people don't get healed? Is it always a lack of faith? What is

---

[85] Capps, 10-11.

our end game with prayer? Sometimes it seems that we think that the only result that is acceptable is healing in this lifetime. The ultimate healing is going to heaven. This life is not our final resting place. At some point, we all must die.

If longevity is the ultimate goal, then the oldest person must be the one most full of faith. But that is not the case. Many young people have died for their faith. Stephen became the first martyr in Acts 7. James, the brother of John, was also martyred. Many have given their life for the faith. I am reminded of one of the most faith-filled people in my lifetime, Kathryn Kuhlman. She had amazing healings during her services, but she was plagued with heart problems. She died on the operating table when she was only 68 years old. These examples tell us that results may be influenced by more than faith. Having said that, let's look at what Jesus said about faith in the next episode.

### Jesus Calms the Storm

The first example shows that Jesus is willing to heal. In the second example, Jesus complements the Centurion for recognizing that He had authority to heal. In this example, Jesus reproves the disciples for not having enough faith.

*23 Then he got into the boat and his disciples followed him.*
*24 Suddenly a furious storm came up on the lake, so that the waves swept over the boat. But Jesus was sleeping. 25 The disciples went and woke him, saying, "Lord, save us! We're going to drown!"*

*26 He replied, "You of little faith, why are you so afraid?" Then he got up and rebuked the winds and the waves, and it was completely calm.*

171

*27 The men were amazed and asked, "What kind of man is this? Even the winds and the waves obey him!"* (Matt. 8:23-27).

This story is amazing. Visualize the drama in this passage because it sets up the next story. Jesus gets in the boat with the disciples. It wasn't a huge boat, but big enough for at least 13 people. Jesus was exhausted from the work of ministry, and He fell asleep. We often forget that Jesus was 100% human and 100% God. The human part was exhausted. How tired do you have to be to fall asleep in a small boat in the middle of a bad storm?

Some of the disciples were seasoned fishermen, who no doubt had seen bad weather while fishing, but this storm scared even them. This storm made the disciples think that they were going to die. "Lord, save us! We're going to drown!" Try to put yourself in the disciples' shoes and consider how you would feel if you thought you were going to drown. The disciples were probably all around 30 years old. All of us tend to think we are bullet proof when we are young. Life usually knocks that out of us at some point. This situation was one of those times.

The disciples did what they should have done. They woke up Jesus. They went to the one that could solve their problem and save their lives. Imagine traveling with Jesus and seeing all the amazing things that He did. In this case, however, before Jesus does anything, He reproves the disciples, "You of little faith, why are you so afraid?" If I was a disciple, I would be thinking, "Don't you see the storm? Look at the boat, we have been bailing water for hours trying to keep it afloat. What do you mean, little faith?"

What was Jesus teaching the disciples...and us at that moment? When you are in the boat with Jesus, the creator of the universe, everything is going to be okay. The disciples and you and I need to trust God in the middle of difficult situations. The Father wants us to trust Him during the storm. In this case, Jesus silenced the storm right away. Often, however, life's challenges go on much longer and require us to trust God much longer. That is where faith is required.

For us to have the faith and trust, we must develop our relationship with the Father. How well do we know God? Do we sense His love? That relationship helps you walk with God through life, through the difficult times.

Faith is also about character. Do we trust that God will do what He says He will do? Do we trust His character? That was the struggle that the 10 spies had after returning from the Promised Land (Num. 13). They didn't believe that God was faithful and would fight for them as they came up against people that were stronger.

When Jesus calmed the storm, the disciples were stunned. They asked the question, "What kind of man is this?" Jesus is more than a man. He is the Son of God and wants to have a relationship with us. In this next story, Jesus once again does the unexpected.

### Jesus Delivers the Demon-Possessed Men

The disciples had a near-death experience and a supernatural encounter with Jesus in the boat. As they landed on the other side of the lake, the unanticipated happens again.

> [28] *When he arrived at the other side in the region of the Gadarenes, two demon-possessed men coming from the tombs met him. They were so violent that no*

173

*one could pass that way.* [29] *"What do you want with us,*
*Son of God?" they shouted. "Have you come here to*
*torture us before the appointed time?"* (Matt. 8:28-29).

Let's stop there to examine a few things. First, the other two gospels record only one demon-possessed man. There are several explanations for that result. I think that the best answer is that the one man was the dominant man, causing him to be noticed more. Don't get hung up on the differences in the accounts. It is common today that when a difficult situation occurs, witnesses often see different aspects of the event. Each person sees things from a different vantage point. A movie called *Vantage Point*, which came out in 2008, highlighted the need to view the assassination attempt on the president from all possible perspectives to get to the truth about what happened. It is the same with Scripture. We need to examine all the evidence available to get to the truth.

The other two gospels, Mark and Luke, give us more details about the situation and how it affected the surrounding communities. They tell us that the local people had attempted to confine the person, even using chains, with no luck. The man had superhuman strength, was totally out of his mind, and couldn't be controlled. But the demons inside of him recognized the authority of Jesus. They begged Him to not torture them. The lesson for us is that the enemy does not have power equal to God. There is no comparison. The demons in Luke's example even begged Jesus to not send them to the Abyss. They know they are defeated and where they will spend eternity.

When the demoniac runs to Jesus and falls at His feet, Jesus asked the demon what was his name, to which he replied, "Legion, for we are many." We don't know anything about how this man got to this way. Was it something that he did or the way he lived? We don't know. We do know that we are told to resist the devil and he will flee from us (James 4). The apostle Peter writes,

> [8] *Be alert and of sober mind. Your enemy the devil prowls around like a roaring lion looking for someone to devour.* [9] *Resist him, standing firm in the faith, because you know that the family of believers throughout the world is undergoing the same kind of sufferings* (1 Pet. 5:8-9).

In Jesus' temptation in Matthew 4, Jesus resists with Scripture. Paul reminds us in Ephesus 6 in his illustration about the full armor of God, that Scripture is a weapon (Eph. 6:17). We need to know God's Word to be able to fight effectively.

As we continue to look at the story of the demoniac, we see that Jesus is faced with a dilemma. What is He going to do with the demons? Watch what He does.

> [30] *Some distance from them a large herd of pigs was feeding.* [31] *The demons begged Jesus, "If you drive us out, send us into the herd of pigs."*
>
> [32] *He said to them, "Go!" So they came out and went into the pigs, and the whole herd rushed down the steep bank into the lake and died in the water.* [33] *Those tending the pigs ran off, went into the town and reported all this, including what had happened to the demon-possessed men.* [34] *Then the whole town went out to meet*

*Jesus. And when they saw him, they pleaded with him to leave their region* (Matt. 8:28-34).

The demons left the man and went into the pigs, and they ran off a steep bank into the lake and drowned. I wonder if Jesus was thinking about the economic loss to the ones that owned the non-kosher pigs. I think that Jesus was thinking about the bigger issue: the restoration of a man to his right mind.

The people from town came out to see what happened. They didn't thank Jesus for helping the man. When they saw the man clothed and in his right mind, Mark records the people as being afraid. They didn't know how to explain the deliverance of this man and the destruction of the pigs. Instead of checking it out and getting to know Jesus, they asked Him to leave. But that is not the end of the story. Both Mark and Luke record the guy that was delivered asking to go with Jesus. Jesus told him to go home and tell his people what the Lord had done for him. I imagine that his family, friends, and neighbors were stunned to see the change.

## CHAPTER 13: MATTHEW 9

### Jesus Heals the Paralyzed Man

This next story shows us how again how someone can intercede for someone else.

*Jesus stepped into a boat, crossed over and came to his own town. ² Some men brought to him a paralyzed man, lying on a mat. When Jesus saw their faith, he said to the man, "Take heart, son; your sins are forgiven."*

*³ At this, some of the teachers of the law said to themselves, "This fellow is blaspheming!"*

*⁴ Knowing their thoughts, Jesus said, "Why do you entertain evil thoughts in your hearts? ⁵ Which is easier: to say, 'Your sins are forgiven,' or to say, 'Get up and walk'? ⁶ But I want you to know that the Son of Man has authority on earth to forgive sins." So he said to the paralyzed man, "Get up, take your mat and go home." ⁷ Then the man got up and went home. ⁸ When the crowd saw this, they were filled with awe; and they praised God, who had given such authority to man* (Matt. 9:1-8).

Both passages tell us that Jesus saw their faith. We get a better understanding of what Jesus saw when we read the account in Mark and Luke. It explains that four men carried the paralyzed man to where Jesus was, but there were so many people that they couldn't get in the house. They didn't give up, but went up on the roof, cut a hole in the roof, and lowered the paralyzed man to where Jesus was. These guys weren't playing around but were going to see their friend healed. The point? Our prayers and actions can work for others.

177

Jesus tells the man to get up and take his mat and go home and he did. The people were amazed. When God works, people are amazed.

## Jesus Raises a Dead Girl and Heals a Sick Woman

These next stories are two of my favorite stories in the Bible because I can visualize them happening. I was in a college choir that performed a musical that presented these two stories in a dramatic fashion. The author of the musical actually came to Arkadelphia, Arkansas and instructed us in how to act out this scene. His instructions embedded this scene in my heart and showed me, for the first time in my life, the power of faith in God.

We can see from the Matthew account that Jesus was talking when a synagogue leader came up to Him to ask for help.

> *[18] While he was saying this, a synagogue leader came and knelt before him and said, "My daughter has just died. But come and put your hand on her, and she will live." [19] Jesus got up and went with him, and so did his disciples"* (Matt. 9:18-19).

Picture this scene: Jesus is teaching with a large crowd around Him. Up walks this guy that Jesus probably doesn't know. He kneels before Jesus and tells Him that his daughter has died. But then he makes a huge confession in the divinity of Jesus. "But come and put your hand on her, and she will live." It doesn't matter what the situation is, Jesus can change the situation. He gives us the possibility of a different outcome. It's true that his daughter was dead, but Jesus could change things. The lesson for us is that it may be true that there is trouble in our life, but Jesus gives us hope when hope is impossible.

The Luke account gives us more information including the synagogue leader's name, Jairus, and his daughter's age, twelve. Luke also tells us that the crowd pressed in on Jesus. That is an important point because it sets up the next part of the scene, the women with bleeding issue.

Jesus doesn't waste any time, but goes with Jairus towards his home. In the middle of the press of the crowd, this desperate woman is determined to reach Jesus. She is weak from her bleeding issue. She isn't even supposed to be there because she is considered unclean, but she is determined to get healed. Luke tells us that she has battled this issue for 12 years, the same amount of time that Jairus's daughter has been alive.

*20 Just then a woman who had been subject to bleeding for twelve years came up behind him and touched the edge of his cloak. 21 She said to herself, "If I only touch his cloak, I will be healed"* (Matt. 9:20).

The gospel of Mark gives us a few more details about the desperation of this women. She spent all her money trying to get help from doctors, but only got worse. When she touches Jesus, Mark records Jesus saying, "Who touched my clothes?" His disciples can't believe Jesus asked the question since the crowd was pressing in on Jesus. Jesus looks around and discovers the woman and she tells Him her story.

*22 Jesus turned and saw her. "Take heart, daughter," he said, "your faith has healed you." And the woman was healed at that moment* (Matt. 9:22).

The woman's faith had healed her. It took twelve years of suffering for her to find her answer in Jesus, but when Jesus showed up, she believed. Faith in Jesus changes things. Her life would never be the same. But the story is not over. Jairus is watching this whole episode. No doubt, he was wanted Jesus to hurry up and help his daughter. Finally, they got going and headed to Jairus' house.

> *²³ When Jesus entered the synagogue leader's house and saw the noisy crowd and people playing pipes, ²⁴ he said, "Go away. The girl is not dead but asleep." But they laughed at him. ²⁵ After the crowd had been put outside, he went in and took the girl by the hand, and she got up. ²⁶ News of this spread through all that region* (Matt. 9:23-26).

People were already mourning the death of this girl. Jesus told them that the girl was not dead but asleep. They laughed at Him. They laughed at the King of Kings and Lord of Lords. They didn't know the power of God was there to heal. I wonder how many times we miss what God wants to do in our lives because we don't believe. When Jesus healed the girl, the word got out. That's what happens when Jesus works in our lives.

## Jesus Heals Two Blind Men and a Mute

When Jesus comes on the scene, word gets out. These two blind men call out to Jesus.

> *²⁷ As Jesus went on from there, two blind men followed him, calling out, "Have mercy on us, Son of David!"*
>
> *²⁸ When he had gone indoors, the blind men came to him, and he asked them, "Do you believe that I am able to do this?"*
>
> *"Yes, Lord," they replied.*

180

*29 Then he touched their eyes and said,*
*"According to your faith let it be done to you"; 30 and*
*their sight was restored. Jesus warned them sternly,*
*"See that no one knows about this." 31 But they went out*
*and spread the news about him all over that region*
(Matt. 9:27-31).

These men were desperate. They weren't afraid of embarrassing themselves in front of people. They wanted help. Often people want God to work in their lives without others knowing about it because it embarrasses them for others to know that they have a need. They are afraid of what people might think about them. These blind men didn't care, they just wanted to be healed. When we go to God, we need to be desperate for God to work in our lives. If it doesn't matter to us, why should it to God?

Jesus asked these men if they believed He could heal them. They said, "Yes." Jesus answered, "According to your faith let it be done to you." As I said before, whether we like it or not, our faith in God matters. Unbelief can affect the outcome of our healing. The next story is a little different.

*32 While they were going out, a man who was*
*demon-possessed and could not talk was brought to*
*Jesus. 33 And when the demon was driven out, the man*
*who had been mute spoke. The crowd was amazed and*
*said, "Nothing like this has ever been seen in Israel."*

*34 But the Pharisees said, "It is by the prince of*
*demons that he drives out demons"* (Matt. 9:32-34).

Jesus says nothing about the mute man's faith. People brought him to Jesus and Jesus healed him. I think that shows the compassion that Jesus has for us when we are struggling. How do we sum up these chapters on healing? I think that God wants us well, but, and that is a big but, I think that we can do things that interfere with our healing. As stated before, how do we treat our body? Do we get enough sleep, eat correctly and exercise? Make changes in these areas. Then, we need to get to know the King of Kings and His Word better. Spend time meditating on God's Word and allow God to reveal himself to you.

As I stated before, I was diagnosed with an incurable cancer almost 9 years ago. I have to trust God every day. At the time of this writing, I am dealing with a lung issue: bronchitis. It is the second time this year. The reason I tell you that is that I am a learner like everyone else. I place my life in the Lord's hands every day. This test makes me think of a passage in James.

> *² Consider it pure joy, my brothers and sisters, whenever you face trials of many kinds, ³ because you know that the testing of your faith produces perseverance. ⁴ Let perseverance finish its work so that you may be mature and complete, not lacking anything* (James 1:2-4).

I know that I talked about this passage earlier, but let me remind you of a couple of things. First, we are to consider it pure joy when we face trials. Why? Because we understand God's purpose: to produce perseverance in us, which is also character change, making us more like Jesus. Let me explain it this way, if I was remodeling my house and you came over to see it before it was done, it might surprise you. The kitchen cabinets are torn down, there is busted sheetrock, and messed up flooring. Everything is dusty and dirty. Of course, it would be obvious to you and anyone else that the process of remodeling the house was underway. You expect things to look bad for a while because you know the end product will be much nicer.

It is the same way with us. God is doing a work in us and when difficulties arise, we are to count it joy because we know that God is remodeling us. So, as you grow in your faith, let Him change you.

# CHAPTER 14: CONCLUSION

There is so much more that could be talked about when discussing faith. As we looked at so many Scriptures, I am convinced that the American church needs more faith. It isn't faith to get more stuff, but more faith to do the work of God. Many Christians don't have a regular plan of growth through Bible study and prayer. As Jesus said, we need to put God first in our lives. We need to lay our lives totally on the Lord, trusting Him to guide us through the challenges we face.

We need to know that God wants to help us in our marriages, with our children, our jobs, our finances, and our health. Christian marriages should be a testimony to the community around us because divorce is so high and the number of those living together is rising. Pew Research Center writes, "The share of adults who have lived with a romantic partner is now higher than the share who have ever been married; married adults are more satisfied with their relationships, more trusting of their partners." [86]

---

[86] Juliana Menasce Horowitz, Nikki Graf, and Gretchen Livingston, "Marriage and Cohabitation in the U.S., Pew Research Center, Washington, D.C., November 6, 2019 https://www.pewresearch.org/social-trends/2019/11/06/marriage-and-cohabitation-in-the-u-s/.

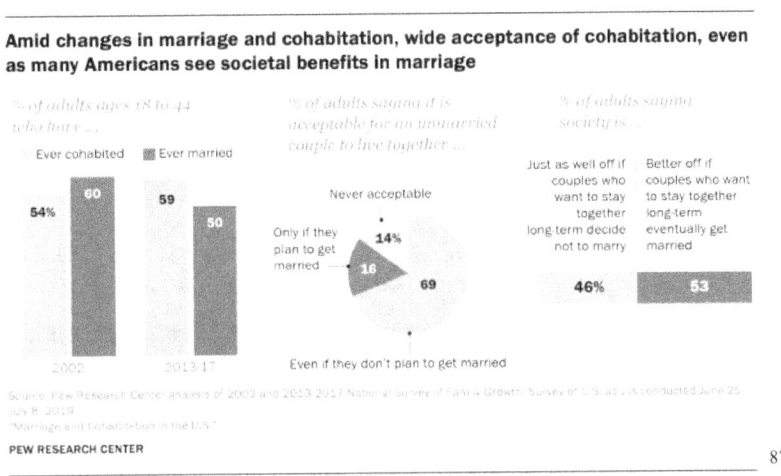

Amid changes in marriage and cohabitation, wide acceptance of cohabitation, even as many Americans see societal benefits in marriage

Source: Pew Research Center analysis of 2002 and 2013-2017 National Survey of Family Growth. Survey of U.S. adults conducted June 25 - July 8, 2019.
"Marriage and Cohabitation in the U.S."

PEW RESEARCH CENTER

The enemy is trying to destroy marriage, churches, and our government. God has an opinion about what we do with our lives. It is exciting to live all out for God. We need to be willing to step out in faith when He calls us to do the impossible. I still don't understand everything about faith, but I do believe that God wants to answer my prayers. I am determined to get to know God better and be open to his leading as well as learning to listen better to His voice.

I trust that you will press into God more and allow Him to challenge you to do more for His kingdom. Step out in faith and see what God does.

Finally, in closing, let me ask you a question. Have you made Jesus Lord and Savior of your life? It is a yes or no question. If you say something like, "I think that I have lived a good life" or "I have done more good than bad," then you don't understand salvation. The Bible tells us that we can

---

[87] Ibid.

know that we are right with God. The Holy Spirit places His earnest payment or down payment on us when we truly accept Jesus as our Lord and Savior. So have you accepted Him as boss of your life. If not, then pray this prayer with me:

*Lord Jesus, I know I am a sinner.*
*I ask you to forgive me of my sins*
*and come into my heart as Lord and Savior of my life.*

That is a simple prayer, but if you meant it, the Holy Spirit places His down payment on you. You should sense his earnest payment in the deepest part of your being. It is important that you get in a good Bible-believing church and begin a regular pattern of Bible study. God bless you in your new adventure.

Bob Ingram

# APPENDIX A: PASTOR BOB'S TESTIMONY

There are so many factors that played into my salvation experience. I will attempt to relate the important and significant pieces of the puzzle that brought me to the beginning of a changed life.

I was raised in an Air Force military family where my dad was an alcoholic, which caused many problems. It could have been worse, but it was bad enough. My mother was a nurse and kept the family together. She took my sister and I to Christian services on the Air Force Base. We listened to sermons, attended Sunday School, later youth group and learned about Jesus. My mother was Lutheran, and when a Lutheran church was built, we attended there. My dad rarely attended church.

During my religious experience through high school, I learned about Jesus, but no one told me that the Bible teaches that salvation comes from accepting Jesus into your heart. If you had asked me if I was a Christian, I would have said something like this, "I believe that I do more good than bad things. I haven't killed anyone, and I don't drink." In another words, I didn't understand salvation. Salvation is a heart change. Salvation involved the grace of God, and we don't work or earn our way to heaven. We accept Jesus into our hearts.

In college, because there was no Lutheran church, I attended other churches. I ended up in a big Southern Baptist church and loved it. I loved the preaching, the Sunday School classes, and, most of all, the college group. During the week, I hung out at the Baptist Student Union where I grew a great deal. But the huge change took place during my 3rd year. I was a music major and played in a jazz band on Friday afternoons. When I finished rehearsal at 5:00, I headed to the cafeteria to eat before it closed. To get to the cafeteria, you walk by the student union. On that night, there were 2 guys wearing jean jackets playing guitars and singing and preaching about Jesus in front of the student union. I was drawn in my spirit to listen to them, but I walked by them. I was embarrassed to listen to the weird guys with long hair and jean jackets playing guitars and singing about Jesus.

Fortunately for me, one of my roommates had accepted Jesus into his heart the previous summer. He must have passed the guys preaching first and decided to turn around. He saw me and encouraged me to go back and listen. To make a long story short, I listened to these guys for 3 hours. They prayed for me to be healed of my bronchitis and I was healed. These guys so moved me that after I left them, I drove my motorcycle way out in the country to find a place to be alone with God. I cried out to God for an hour. I gave Him my entire life, including my motorcycle. You know that you are serious about God when you give Him your prized possession: your motorcycle. If you asked me after that night if I was a Christian, I would have said "yes" because of what Jesus did for me. There was no doubt Jesus was Lord of my life.

Things began to happen. I became a Baptist summer missionary to Baltimore, Maryland for 10 weeks. I learned a bunch there, but the main thing I learned was that I needed more of Jesus. I prayed two prayers, one to use my music for God and the other to have more of Him. God answered both prayers. I joined a gospel group based out of an Interdenominational church. This church was phenomenal and greatly changed my life. They taught me about the Bible and encouraged me to study it. They fasted and prayed and read and memorized the Scriptures and hugged each other. They were crazy, but it changed me. I started memorizing Scriptures and meditating on them. Also, got I got more of Jesus: I was filled with the Holy Spirit.

I would stay with this church and the gospel group until a car wreck took me out. Over the next four months, I recovered from the car wreck and sought the Lord. Eventually, God led me to the Teen Challenge ministry where I would work for 4 years and meet my future wife, Dana, who also worked there. Today, we have been married 47 years and have two daughters, two sons-in-law, and two grandkids. I am a blessed man.

Much more could be said about my conversion experience. When I got saved, I got saved. It was deep-seated, and my life was changed. How do I know that? The car wreck that took me out of the gospel group showed me. I rolled the car over 6 times and was knocked out. When I came to, a guy was standing over me looking down at me. He was the guy with whom I almost had the head-on collision. After he passed me, he turned around and came back, and I was still knocked out.

When I woke up, he asked me if he could pray for me. Before he prayed for me, I could remember my name, someone was with me going somewhere, and that Jesus was Lord of my life. My salvation experience was deep-seated all the way to the core of my being. That was that earnest payment about which Paul talks.

*[13] And you also were included in Christ when you heard the message of truth, the gospel of your salvation.*

*When you believed, you were <u>marked in him with a seal,</u>
<u>the promised Holy Spirit,</u> [14] who is a <u>deposit</u>
<u>guaranteeing</u> our inheritance until the redemption of
those who are God's possession—to the praise of his
glory* (Eph. 1:13-14).

Deep inside of me, I knew that I belonged to God. I carry that knowledge with me all the time and everywhere. I hope that you can have that same deep-seated experience of accepting Jesus into your life. If you don't know Him, you can fix that by asking Jesus to forgive you of your sins and to come into your heart as Lord and Savior. Often people want the Savior part without the Lord part. It takes both. Jesus needs to be Lord, ruler, and boss of your life. If you make that decision to accept Jesus as Lord and Savior, your sins are forgiven, and you will spend eternity with Jesus in heaven.

Once you accept Jesus into your heart, you need to get in a Bible-believing church and begin studying the Bible. You will learn how to live for God. It is a wonderful adventure and I have never regretted giving my life to Jesus.

# APPENDIX B: PASTOR BOB'S ADVENTURE INTO AVIATION

My dad was a WWII fighter pilot. He flew P-51s and P-38s, two of the most capable aircraft during their time. But for several reasons, he got out of flying but stayed in the Air Force. I heard a little bit of my dad's war history, but he didn't talk about flying much. My dad stayed in the Air Force until a heart attack medically retired him after almost 26 years of service. We were stationed around the country and overseas. We lived on the military bases sometimes and off base at other times, but I was always close to airplanes. Even though I saw airplanes all the time, I never thought about flying them. In fact, I was in Civil Air Patrol in high school and flew a few times in small airplanes, but it didn't interest me. I knew I couldn't fly in the military because I wore glasses, so flying was never much of a thought to me.

I went to college on a music scholarship, graduated and played with a gospel group. A car wreck took me out of the group. While looking for a job, I worked at Wal-Mart. During my prayer time, the Lord told me He would put me in full-time ministry. I said "okay" but applied for teaching jobs. I was laid off after Christmas from Wal-Mart. A friend invited me to come to a New Year's Eve service at Teen Challenge of Little Rock. Since I didn't have a job, I went. During the service, the Lord laid the burden of Teen Challenge on my life.[88] I knew little about the program, only that God

---

[88] Teen Challenge is a Christian drug rehab program started by David Wilkerson around 1960. Today it has programs all over the country and around the world.

called me there. My future wife, Dana, was already working for Teen Challenge. We would meet and be married in a little over a year and are now, at the time of this writing, on our 48th year of marriage.

During my fourth year at Teen Challenge, I turned on the TV and saw a Cessna "Learn to fly commercial". I felt drawn in my spirit to check this out. Never in my wildest imagination did I think I would ever fly for a living. I didn't have the time, money, or desire to learn to fly. But I was obedient and set up a flying lesson 60 miles away in Fort Smith, Arkansas. There wasn't even an airport close by because we were so far back in the woods. By now, I was running the younger boy's program in Northwest Arkansas. The big town was 13 miles away and had only something over 1000 people.

I asked the Lord to confirm His will to me and He did. A guy had regularly come out to the boy's center to do some electrical work for us. One day, I told him I was going to take a flying lesson. He perked up and said, "From whom?" I told him and he said, "Why don't you take lessons from me? I am an instructor, and I won't even charge you." "Are you sure?", I asked. "Well, you can pay me for the airplane when you have the money." I felt that was confirmation.

As soon as I began flying, it was different than before. It was a passion. There was never a day I was tired of flying. I got tired of other things involved in the business of flying, but not flying. I enjoyed the systems knowledge and the troubleshooting. Dealing with weather and instrument approaches constantly challenged me. I flew for a living for 31 years until God took me to the next chapter.

There is much more to the story, but know this: what God wants for you, He will provide for you and direct you if you will be obedient and step out in faith.

# SOURCES CONSULTED

Arnason, Terra G., Matthew W. Bowen and Kerry D. Nansell. "Effects of intermittent fasting on health markers in those with type 2 diabetes: A pilot study World Journal of Diabetes" in National Library of Medicine: National Center for Biotechnical Information. April 15, 2017. https://www.ncbi.nlm.nih.gov/pmc/articles/PMC5394735/.

Barclay, William. *The Letters of James and Peter* in *The New Daily Study Bible*. Revised Edition. Louisville, KY: Westminster John Knox Press, 1975.

Blomberg, Craig. *Matthew, The New American Commentary*, Vol. 22. Nashville: Broadman & Holman Publishers, 1992.

Bonhoeffer, Dietrich. *The Cost of Discipleship*. Translated by Chr. Kaiser Verlag Munchen, R.H. Fuller, and Irmgard Booth. New York: Touchstone, 1995.

Brooks, James A. *Mark, The New American Commentary*, Vol. 23. Nashville: Broadman & Holman Publishers, 1991.

Capps, Charles. *The Tongue, A Creative Force*. Tulsa, OK: Harrison House, 1976.

Colwell, Abby and Sun Eoh, Megan Halpern, and Kate Shea. "Stone-Hurling Catapult, Greece 400BCE." Smith College Museum of Ancient Inventions, 1997-1998. https://www.smith.edu/hsc/museum/ancient_inventions/hsc11b.htm.

Cooper, Rodney L. *Mark, Holman New Testament Commentary*, Vol. 2. Nashville: Broadman & Holman Publishers, 2000.

Elliott, Mickey. "Understanding the 10 Commandments and their relevance for today." Reporter-Times. December 10, 2021. https://www.reporter-times.com/story/lifestyle/faith/2021/12/10/understanding-10-commandments-and-their-relevance-today/6457925001/.

Ferguson, Shani. "Seven ways Israel has impacted your world. Kehila News. July 12, 2018. https://news.kehila.org/seven-ways-israel-has-impacted-your-world/.

Foster, Richard J. *Celebration of Discipline: The Path to Spiritual Growth*. New York: HarperOne, 1998.

Geldenhuys, Norval. *The Gospel of Luke, The International Commentary on the New Testament*. Grand Rapids, MI: W.M. B. Eerdmans Publishing Co. Reprinted, 1988.

Got Questions.org. "*About Got Questions.Org*." Accessed October 14, 2022. https://www.gotquestions.org/about.html.

Got Questions.org. "What does the Bible say about the prosperity gospel?". Accessed October 14, 2022. https://www.gotquestions.org/prosperity-gospel.html.

Got Questions.org. "What is the difference between faith and hope?". Accessed October 15,2022. https://www.gotquestions.org/difference-faith-hope.html.

Hackett, Conrad, and David McClendon. "Christians remain world's largest religious group, but they are declining in Europe." April 5, 2017. https://www.pewresearch.org/fact-tank/2017/04/05/christians-remain-worlds-largest-religious-group-but-they-are-declining-in-europe/.

Harrison, Everett F. *Introduction to the New Testament*. Grand Rapids, MI: WM. B. Eerdmans, 1982.

Hill, Napoleon. *Think and Grow Rich: The Landmark Bestseller—Now Revised and Updated for the 21st Century* by Arthur R. Pell. New York: Jeremy P. Tarcher/Penguin, 2005.

Horowitz, Juliana Menasce, Nikki Graf and Gretchen Livingston. "Marriage and Cohabitation in the U.S." Pew Research Center. November 6, 2019. https://www.pewresearch.org/social-trends/2019/11/06/marriage-and-cohabitation-in- the-u-s/.

Jackson, Gloria Beech. *Through the Fire: Suffering as an Integral Component of Christian Life and Ministry*. Springfield, MO: Life Publishers International, 2011.

Jones, David W. "5 Errors of the Prosperity Gospel." The Gospel Coalition. June 5, 2015. https://www.thegospelcoalition.org/article/5-errors-of-the-prosperity-gospel/.

Jones, David W., and Russell S. Woodbridge. *Health, Wealth, and Happiness: How the Prosperity Gospel Overshadows the Gospel of Christ*. Grand Rapids, MI: Kregel Publications, 2017.

Jones, Jeffery M. "Belief in God in U.S. Dips to 81%, a New Low." Gallup.com. June 17, 2022. https://news.gallup.com/poll/393737/belief-god-dips-new-low.aspx.

Morris, Leon. *Luke: An Introduction and Commentary, Tyndale New Testament Commentaries,* vol. 3. Downers Grove, IL: InterVarsity Press. 1988.

Nelson Mandela Foundation. "Biography of Nelson Mandela." Accessed Dec. 19, 2022. https://www.nelsonmandela.org/content/page/biography

Purkiser, W.T. ed., C.E. Damaray, Donald S. Metz, and Maude A. Stuneck. *Exploring the Old Testament*. Kansas City, MO: Beacon Hill Press, 1955.

Richter, Amy and Rachael Ajmera. "8 Health Benefits of Fasting, Backed by Science." Healthline, March 13, 2023. https://www.healthline.com/nutrition/fasting-benefits.

Robert Tilton Ministries. "How to be Rich and Have Everything You Always Wanted." Accessed October 16, 2022. https://store.aegispremier.com/wof/product/Download/DWBK-01.

Rowett, Amanda. "The Prison of Unforgiveness: A Christian Counselor's Perspective on Forgiveness." Bellevue Christian Counseling. April 14, 2015; https://bellevuechristiancounseling.com/articles/the-prison-of-unforgiveness

Schreiner, Thomas R. *1,2 Peter, Jude*, Vol. 37, *The New American Commentary*. Nashville: Broadman & Holman Publishers, 2003.

Schultz, Samuel J. *The Old Testament Speaks: A Complete Survey of Old Testament History and Literature*, 4th ed. San Francisco: Harper and Row, 1990.

Sobel, Dava. *Longitude: The True Story of a Lone Genius Who Solved the Greatest Scientific Problem of His Time*. London: Fourth Estate Limited, 1998.

Strassner, Kurt. *Opening up Genesis*. Leominster, England: Day One Publication, 2009.

Tenney, Merrill C. *New Testament Times*. 1965. Grand Rapids, MI: Williams B. Eerdmans Publishing Company, Sixth printing, 1978.

Willard, Dallas. *The Divine Conspiracy: Rediscovering Our Hidden Life in God*. New York, NY: HarperCollins Publishers, 1998.

Weber, Jeremy. "Surprising Starts on Who Reads the Bible from Start to Finish." ChristianityToday.com. June 4, 2013. https://www.christianitytoday.com/news/2013/june/surprising-stats-on-who-reads-bible-from-start-to-finish.html.

Wikipedia. "Robert Tilton." Accessed March 27, 2023. https://en.wikipedia.org/wiki/Robert_Tilton.

Wilkerson, David. *The Vision: A Terrifying Prophecy of Doomsday That is Starting to Happen Now*. Spire Books, 1973.

Zwick, Edward, director. *The Last Samurai*. Warner Bros. Pictures, 2003. https://en.wikipedia.org/wiki/The_Last_Samurai.

www.ingramcontent.com/pod-product-compliance
Lightning Source LLC
Chambersburg PA
CBHW070542220526
45467CB00003B/1023